STRONG TO THE CORE

STRONG TO THE CORE

Get on the ball for a strong, lean physique

LISA WESTLAKE

AURUM PRESS

First published in the United Kingdom 2003 by
Aurum Press Limited, 25 Bedford Avenue, London WC1B 3AT

Produced by ABC Books for
The Australian Broadcasting Corporation

A catalogue record for this book is available from the British Library

ISBN 1 85410 947 2

2007	2006	2005	2004
5	4	3	2

Designed by Ingo Voss, vossdesign
Set in 9/11.75 Rotis semi serif
Colour seperation by Colorwize Studio, Adelaide
Printed and bound in Singapore by Tien Wah Press

The exercises and advice given in this book are in no way intended as a substitute for
medical advice and guidance. Consult your doctor before beginning this or any other
exercise program. The author and publisher take no responsibility for any injury that
may be caused as a result of applying the information in this book.

dedication

To dear friends who left too early - Lou, Barb and Kate, this is for you.

contents

strong to the core

Are you willing to raise your training to higher levels of quality using innovative concepts and a fresh approach for the ultimate reward - a strong, defined physique and a body that looks fantastic and is truly fit for living?

Whether you are an elite athlete, a regular gym-goer or a determined beginner, training with an exercise ball can provide fantastic results.

Strong to the core is a comprehensive guide to working-out with this revolutionary fitness tool. It provides innovative and effective exercise techniques for strength training, back health and injury prevention. This book is for those seeking muscle tone and definition but who also want a stronger, healthier, injury-free body.

Strong to the core will help you achieve the very best from your exercise ball. Proud posture, defined muscle tone and deep abdominal stability are just a few of the benefits you'll see and feel.

Enjoy the workout — you'll love the results!

Using an exercise ball for strength and fitness may be a relatively new concept, but it is not just another fitness fad. The ball has been used extensively in rehabilitation and physiotherapy for more than 30 years. The idea of broadening its use from a strictly medical rehabilitation device to a mainstream fitness tool came about in the early 1990s. It is now extremely popular in gyms, for personal training and for home programs. Sporting clubs and trainers recognise its value for injury prevention, sport-specific training and improved athletic performance.

This is a training tool that is here to stay.

Basic exercise ball principles, combined with strength conditioning, provide an exceptional workout, above and beyond other more expensive, cumbersome or complicated routines and equipment.

Simple principles. Simple equipment. Sensational results.

so, why train on an exercise ball?

apart from the fabulous physical benefits ... here's why!

Variety

If you've been training for a while now, you may be finding yourself in an 'exercise comfort zone'. You cruise through the same old workout, possibly several days per week. You're keeping fit but are you really getting the best out of your regular ritual? New motivation and interest come from added challenge and a fresh approach to old favourites introduced by using an exercise ball.

Challenge

Basically the ball is 'wobbly' so you will draw on extra muscles and develop new skills. Several more outer and deep muscles are recruited when training on the ball, some of which you may never have felt before. Simply sitting on it will have you working harder to perform upper body strengthening.

Improved technique

It is often alarming to see people using incorrect technique while training. Apart from the fact they are cheating on their workout, sloppy technique means they are also placing their bodies at risk.

By working on the exercise ball you will automatically, often subconsciously, correct and improve your exercise quality. If you lose good posture, the ball will roll or wobble, prompting you to correct your form.

Physical benefits

Working out on an exercise ball has a variety of physical benefits – from gentle stretching, to intense strengthening – for young and old, and all levels of fitness. They include:

- **Back health** — strengthens the structures directly responsible for spinal health and injury prevention.

- **Improved posture** — the act of balancing builds postural awareness and strength.

- **Core stability** — basically this means that your deep abdominal and spinal muscles – which act as a splint around your spine – are worked and therefore strengthened.

- **Muscle balance** — 'reversing' muscle imbalances, which can cause back injuries and postural problems.

- **Mobility and flexibility** — to relax, release and rejuvenate your whole body.

back in action

And it's a sad fact that regular exercise can't guarantee you a pain-free back for life. Even fit and obviously strong people remain vulnerable to back injury. In fact, poor exercise choices and incorrect technique can actually place the gym-goer at higher risk.

So shouldn't our training regimes be modified to focus as much on posture and injury prevention as fitness?

Absolutely!

Back pain can be caused by several factors.

Stiffness
Poor postures and prolonged positions associated with daily life and work — such as sitting at a desk — can cause immobility, stiffness and weakness.

Muscle imbalances
Daily activities and inappropriate exercise can lead to muscle imbalances, therefore increasing the risk of postural problems and back pain.

Deep weakness
Core stability is the missing link between exercise and the prevention of back pain. Weakness and poor function of the deep, stabilising muscles are closely associated with back pain and injury. Yet, until recently, the role played by these 'bracing' muscles has not been fully appreciated.

Tightness

Certain muscles that are overused, or constantly resting in their shortened position, become tight and pull our bodies out of alignment.

Stress and overloading

Fast movements, sudden twisting and heavy lifting are all notorious for causing back pain in everyday activities and during exercise.

Most back pain is the result of a combination of instability, poor posture and the activities of daily life gradually contributing to a weakened and vulnerable spine.

The spine is a complex, hard-working structure. For injury-prevention, we need more than is offered in traditional workouts. The exercise ball routines set out in Strong to the core incorporate core stability, mobility, muscle balance, and flexibility to strengthen your back against injury.

So whether you've suffered a back problem in the past or you want to prevent injury for the future, these exercises will help you achieve a stronger, healthier back.

Strong to the core unites health, fitness and injury-prevention, promoting a workout that will not only have you looking and feeling great, but that will also keep you mobile, flexible, balanced and fit for living.

posture

good posture is when your spine is in natural alignment

Natural spinal curves play an important role in the health of your back.

Standing in front of a mirror, you will notice your lower back is not flat, but has a slight sway. When your back is in this **neutral spine alignment**, the ligaments, muscles and discs are at their optimal position and under the least stress.

For a healthy back, aim to maintain this neutral spine during daily activities and exercise.

Hint: Think long spine rather than straight back.

Particularly relevant to exercise ball training is what is called the **lumbar lordosis** – the slight sway of the lower back. The aim is to maintain this curve, and not to let it either increase or flatten out. In the past we were encouraged to flatten our backs, particularly while doing abdominal curls. This was an attempt to protect the spine from stress during exercise, but we now know this is not ideal from a technical point of view.

Rather, maintaining your natural lumbar curve is best practice. In fact, attention to your whole spine will help minimise discomfort and injury, while improving exercise benefits. Try to keep your neck in line with your spine, your shoulder blades set back and down (avoid the hunching that sometimes accompanies exercise effort) and your spine long and in natural curvature.

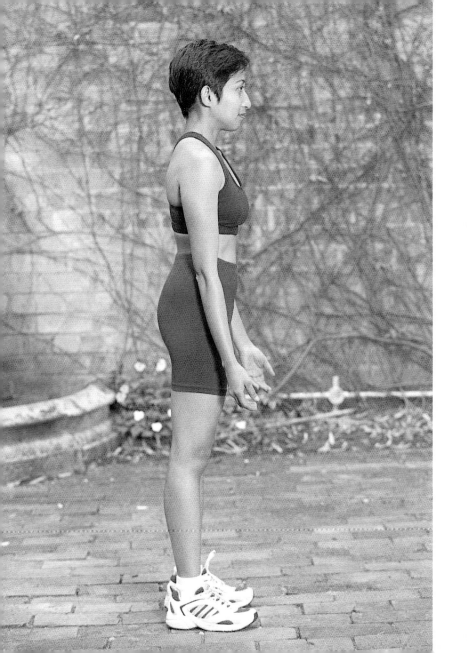

core stability

so what is core stability, and why are deep muscles that we can't even feel so important?

The muscles responsible for supporting the spine are the spinal stabilisers. More specifically, the deep abdominals and deep back muscles stabilise and support the lower-back area.

Until recently these have been considered out of sight, out of mind. However, new research has demonstrated how vital they are to maintaining core stability. Understanding the importance of core control brings a new meaning to total body conditioning.

Core control is the ability of specific deep muscles to brace and support the spine, shoulder or pelvis. Probably the most thoroughly investigated and best understood is stabilisation of the lower back.

Research has demonstrated that healthy deep abdominal and back muscles contract to 'splint' the lumbar vertebrae, providing support for movement such as throwing, lifting or running. In fact, these deep muscles are required to support virtually every movement, even those that are not heavy or extreme. Without adequate stabilisation, the risk of injury rises.

For a number of years we recommended abdominal curls to help your back. We now know that although we were on the right track, we were focusing on the wrong muscles. The outer abdominals — such as those used in curls — can be trained for strength and definition, but play no role in spinal stability.

The muscles responsible for supporting the lumbar spine are the deepest abdominal muscle (**transversus abdominus**) and the deepest back muscle (**multifidus**), in conjunction with other muscles such as the **internal obliques**. These muscles work together like a low belt or corset around the spine. When they fail to function effectively, the lower back is unsupported and vulnerable to injury.

Moreover, the pelvic floor works in conjunction with the deep abdominals. So, any exercise that strengthens the deep stabilising muscles also improves pelvic floor control and vice versa. This is of benefit to everyone, especially those prone to incontinence.

These core muscles are hard to feel, impossible to see and do not create movement, so it can be hard to recognise them initially. But with time and practice you will become more aware of the stabilisers and notice the difference they provide to exercise and daily life. Contracting the deep abdominals correctly is an integral component of this program and is taught on page 26.

So, if you're just beginning a fitness regime, get on the ball and combine core strength with outer conditioning, right from the start.

And if you already train, it's time to add this deep dimension to your workout. Improved core stabilisation not only protects you from injury, it will also have you standing taller and looking stronger and it will provide you with the deep strength to take your training, sport and physical life to higher levels.

muscle balance

Traditional strength programs tend to focus on **anterior** muscles – those in the front of our bodies, which we see when looking straight at a mirror. Even without specific training, these muscles are stronger than their opposing **posterior** groups because they are the main muscles used to push, pull and perform other daily activities. The posterior muscles, however, are the ones required for tall, upright posture.

All muscles groups have an opposing muscle – biceps and triceps are an example. If the anterior muscle is stronger than its posterior counterpart, muscle imbalance occurs. There is a tendency for the stronger muscle to be tighter. In relation to the torso, this compromises posture. Over time this can create problems such as slouching, stooping or a sway back. Apart from being unhealthy for the spine, these are not good looks!

Unfortunately, traditional weight training programs don't help when they favour exercises that strengthen anterior muscle groups, such as push-ups, abdominal curls and bench presses.

So why do people naturally prefer to train these front muscles, since they are already stronger? There are several reasons.

Firstly, 'mirror muscle syndrome'. If our reason for training is even partly appearance, it is not surprising that we focus on muscles we can see.

Secondly, because these muscles are stronger they are more gratifying and satisfying to use in a workout.

Finally, training the posterior counterparts is often awkward.

Overtraining anterior muscles and neglecting the important posterior postural muscles only aggravates muscle imbalances, increasing the likelihood of poor posture and injury. For healthy backs and sensational physiques, our natural anterior muscle strength should be balanced with more emphasis on posterior muscle groups.

Admittedly, it can be difficult to find positions and actions that are safe and effective for strengthening these back muscles. Old-fashioned options had us leaning forward in difficult, unsafe positions, or lying on the floor with little room to move.

But the ball provides an elegant, efficient solution. When lying prone (forward) over the ball, the lower back is supported while the body is off the floor. This gives the arms and legs adequate space and range of movement to perform effective strengthening routines for the upper back, shoulder girdle, lower back and buttocks.

mobility and flexibility

to truly optimise the health of your body and mind, give
mobility and flexibility the time and respect they deserve

Sometimes forgotten, but extremely important aspects of health and fitness are mobility
of the joints and flexibility of the muscles. Joint stiffness and tight muscles create
limitations in movement and compromise posture. Both can contribute to pain and
the risk of injury.

The natural flow and motion of an exercise ball can be used to mobilise, stretch and relax
your body, preventing muscle tightness and joint stiffness. In turn, this improves your
quality of movement and decreases the risk of injury.

Every strength exercise in Strong to the core has a complementary stretch, which is
identified for your convenience. You may choose to stretch after each exercise or you
may like to complete your training with a combination of stretches. Use the flexibility
section for post-exercise stretching or on its own for a gentle 'mind/body' session.
There are also a specific flexibility training programs (pages 172 and 173).

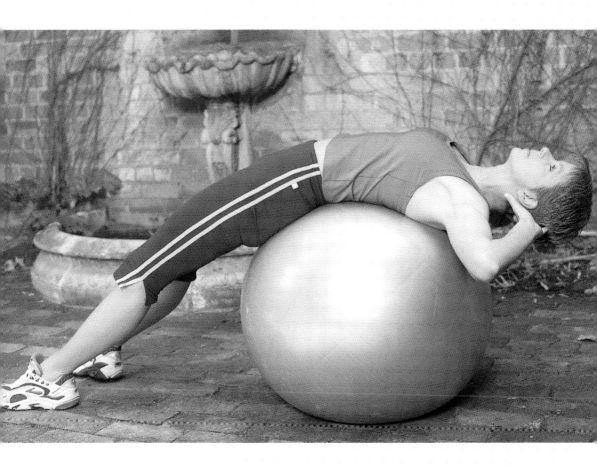

exercise ball principles

so what is it about an oversized ball that makes it such an effective and versatile fitness tool? How can such a simple device reap such diverse rewards?

There are several basic principles at work here:
- instability
- mobility
- lever length
- positioning

Instability

A ball workout combines an unstable base of support (the ball) and a stable base of support (the floor). Exercising on an unstable base activates your deepest abdominal muscles (core stability), balance and proprioception (body awareness).

Using different positions allows you to work on stabilising and strengthening different parts of your body. For example, sitting on the ball with your feet on the floor trains lumbar (lower back) stability, while lying in the forward prone position with your legs on the ball and your hands on the floor requires stabilisation of the shoulder girdle and spine.

Performing a full range of exercises on the ball optimises back health and leads to higher levels of performance in training and daily life.

Different degrees of stability, balance and levels of challenge are provided by simply altering the base of support, the centre of gravity, weight load or lever length. For example, you can start the seated exercises with your feet hip-width apart. Simply bringing them closer together (narrowing your base of support) will increase the challenge.

Mobility
The fact that the ball moves easily means that it rolls if you lose good form and posture. This instant feedback makes you automatically improve exercise technique.

The mobility of the ball also creates a wonderful flow of movement, making it ideal for facilitating joint mobility and flexibility.

Lever length
In many of the exercises throughout Strong to the core you can alter the lever length – the distance of the 'load' (your body) from the 'fulcrum' (the point at which your body is balancing on the ball) – to increase or decrease intensity.

For example, to do a push-up in the forward prone position the ball is under your legs and your hands are on the ground. To lengthen the lever and increase the challenge, walk your hands out until the ball is under your toes. To shorten the lever and decrease the challenge, you can walk back until it is under your thighs.

Positioning
The fact that the ball is portable and mobile means it provides a wonderful base for exercise positioning. You can sit on it and lie forward, backwards and sideways on it. You can rest your back against it and you can lie on the floor and rest your legs on it. Some people can even kneel and stand on the ball, although this is only appropriate for experienced exercisers at an elite level.

Exercising in all positions that the ball allows will provide you with many advantages over using a chair or bench, such as improved posture, extra muscle recruitment and increased challenge.

the truth
about exercise

While gazing in awe at a person with ultimate tone and definition, take a moment
to realise this has not happened overnight. Dedication and effort have gone into
that body you're admiring.

Patience, good sense and plenty of determination will get you there, too.

And although an exercise ball is undoubtedly an excellent tool for building strength
and stability, other aspects of health and fitness must complement your efforts to
help you reach your ultimate goal.

These include:
- a sensible diet
- adequate hydration
- quality sleep
- rest and relaxation
- regular cardiovascular exercise
- strength
- flexibility
- variety

Achieving a fit, lean body requires a combination of exercise, healthy eating, common
sense and dedication. Remember too that time, a sense of commitment and setting
realistic goals are also essential.

All these factors come together to create great results – and if you need assistance
in any of these areas, seek advice from an appropriate professional.

A healthy diet is the most important place to start. There are numerous diets around, but at the end of the day if you are eating a high proportion of fresh, healthy, colourful food and a low proportion of processed or junk food, you will always be on the right track.

If excess body fat is hiding your muscular development, a combination of the right exercise and a varied diet should help you look as strong as you feel. A professional dietitian will be able to advise you further about healthy eating and weight loss.

Cardiovascular exercise is probably the next most important element of a strength and fitness plan and is an indispensable accompaniment to working out on the ball. Regularly performing both will further boost the fitness of your heart, lungs and circulation.

Doing between 20 and 40 minutes of cardiovascular exercise (anything that makes you puff, such as walking, running, swimming and cycling) three to four times a week will help you feel fitter, lose weight and increase your energy.

If time is an issue, introduce some incidental exercise into your day to get you started. For example, use the stairs instead of the escalator or lift, park your car a little further away from your destination, or walk with the kids to school.

To learn more about cardio training, consult a qualified fitness professional.

The best time for your cardiovascular routine is either before doing the ball exercises in Strong to the core, or on alternating days.

how heavy?

work out with weights on the ball to build strength and core stability

Because certain muscle groups are stronger than others, you need two or three different levels of weights. As your strength increases, gradually increase the load.

Obviously people of different ages, fitness levels and degrees of previous experience require varying weights.

To help you choose the right weight for any particular exercise, we have called them

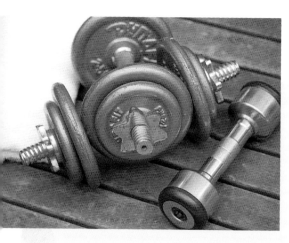

Level 1 (light)
Level 2 (medium)
Level 3 (heavy)

Use the table to guide you in your choice of weights and to recognise when it's time to progress.

If you're already used to working with weights on terra firma, you may need to go a few sizes lighter to start with. Regular conditioning exercises are much harder to do with good form on the exercise ball than on a stable base.

Even if you now have good external muscle strength, your core control muscles may need a little time to catch up. Be patient, always focus on quality not quantity and you will soon be increasing your weights again. Remember, taking the time to strengthen these foundations will ultimately take your strength and training further.

EXPERIENCE/ STRENGTH	LEVEL 1	LEVEL 2	LEVEL 3
BACK, NECK OR SHOULDER PAIN INJURED, PREGNANT	NO WEIGHTS	NO WEIGHTS	NO WEIGHTS
STARTING OUT ON THE BALL NO WEIGHT TRAINING EXPERIENCE	NO WEIGHTS	NO WEIGHTS	2.5 LB/1 KG
MINIMAL EXPERIENCE ON BALL OR WITH WEIGHTS	NO WEIGHTS	2.5 LB/1KG	5 LB/2 KG
COMFORTABLE WITH BASIC BALL EXERCISES OR WORKED A LITTLE WITH WEIGHTS	2.5LB/1 KG	5 LB/2 KG	7 LB/3 KG
CONFIDENT ON THE BALL AND WORKED WITH WEIGHTS	5 LB/2 KG	7 LB/2KG	10 LB/4 KG
OFTEN WORKS WITH WEIGHTS BUT LITTLE EXPERIENCE ON THE BALL	5 LB/2 KG	7 LB/2 KG	10 LB/4 KG
EXPERIENCE WITH WEIGHTS AND BALL TRAINING	7 LB/3 KG	10 LB/4 KG	12-15 LB/5-6 KG

HINTS

IF VERY HEAVY MUSCLE TRAINING IS YOUR PASSION, COMBINING STRENGTH TRAINING ON AND OFF THE BALL WILL BOOST YOUR PROGRAM. USE LIGHTER WEIGHTS FOR A FEW SETS ON THE BALL, THEN A HEAVY SET ON A FIRM BASE SUCH AS A BENCH OR THE GROUND.

WHILE FEELING YOUR MUSCLES BURN WHEN YOU WORK MAY BE YOUR GOAL, BE SURE TO DIFFERENTIATE THIS FROM PAIN RELATING TO JOINT STRESS OR EXCESSIVE INTENSITY. DO NOT CONTINUE ANY EXERCISE THAT CAUSES PAIN.

how many?

Everybody is different, so to quantify specific numbers or repetitions is limiting. Sets and repetitions are suggested for each exercise as a guide only.

For example, two sets of 15 (15 x 2) means to do the exercise 15 times, have a brief rest, then do another 15 repetitions (reps).

Experienced weight-trainers know there are many approaches when it comes to reps and sets, but keep in mind that exercising on the ball is well suited to lower resistance and higher repetition. This builds endurance.

If you are interested in exploring different training methods, use the exercises in this book with an experienced personal trainer. And for optimal results without injury, always place the quality of what you do well above the quantity.

how long?

Workouts should last from 30 minutes to an hour depending on your exercise and program selection and your level of fitness. As you become fitter and stronger you'll find you can increase your workout time and intensity.

Aim to do Strong to the core exercises three to four times per week and combine these with other favourite exercise options. This cross-training will keep you motivated and will provide the variety your body needs to keep improving.

Vary your training focus to avoid stress and repetition on any muscle group. Plenty of diversity and two or three days of rest each week will ensure you don't overdo it and keep you injury-free.

Choose exercises from Strong to the core to customise your own workout or select any of the programs on pages 166 to 183.

exercise technique

good form and movement control will make or break a training program.

By paying attention to sound technique and efficient posture you will reap the best results.

Always make sure you are in good position while on the ball (use a mirror if possible), and concentrate on moving slowly and smoothly through every exercise. Avoid jolting or swinging. Pay attention to how well you are moving at the same time as holding your body and the ball stable.

You should stay in control of the movement. If you are wobbling or losing form, lighten the load. Remember, the aim is to build quality before you start increasing quantity.

You'll eventually get further, faster if you focus on control and quality at all times.

what you need

The only equipment you need for your ball workout is:
- the right exercise ball for your height
- hand weights, ideally two or three different pairs
- a safe, non-slip space
- a mat or towel for when you lie on the floor
- time! For best results, try for 30 to 60 minutes, three to four times per week.

increasing
the challenge

if you want results you need to challenge your body

You'll know you're working at the right level if the last few reps of an exercise feel tough, but you are still maintaining excellent form.

Once you notice you're completing an exercise with ease and good form, you are ready to progress.

To increase the challenge, you can adjust:
- load/weights
- repetitions and/or sets
- instability (base of support)
- length of lever

A general approach to increasing intensity is to add an extra few reps to each set, perform an extra set or increase your weights. Likewise, you can decrease your effort by lightening the load, performing fewer reps or deleting a set.

Remember that when you increase your weights you are increasing the challenge to your core stability as well as your outer prime moving muscles. If you are starting to cheat or lose technique, shake or feel pain, you are overdoing it. This compromises your form and safety and will not produce your desired results.

Fine tune your workout by listening to your body and carefully assessing how you feel at the end of the suggested number of reps and sets.

but take care

Always consult a health professional before beginning any exercise program. Certain exercises on the ball are highly effective for people such as pregnant women or those with back pain. In the custom designed programs on pages 170 to 173 you will find specific regimes for back health and pre-natal exercise.

It is important to realise, however, that other exercise ball options are inappropriate for people with special needs. If you have an injury, illness, disability or are pre- or post-natal, it is especially important that you consult with your physiotherapist or health professional to assess whether the exercises in Strong to the core are suitable for you and to guide you in selecting safe and appropriate exercises.

Although the exercise ball was initially used in therapy, this book is not intended for rehabilitation or injury management and should not be used to replace treatment or manual therapy.

Safety tips
- avoid using the exercise ball on slippery surfaces
- keep your distance from sharp objects, heaters and steps
- stop any exercise that causes discomfort

setting the abdominals

setting the abdominals plays an important role in all types of exercise, but even more so when it comes to exercising on the ball

When you work out on the ball, you constantly switch on your core muscles to hold your back long, to maintain neutral lumbar curve and to keep your back, and the ball, still. So correct technique is vital and deserves special attention.

You need to activate the stabilising muscles by setting the abdominals in virtually every exercise. You should not progress with your ball work or increase the challenge of any exercise until you establish good core control. Practise the setting action as an important preliminary step.

Sitting tall on the ball, place one hand in the small of your back. Notice the natural lumbar curve. Now place your second hand on your lower abdomen, below your naval. The deep abdominals lie beneath this area. Lengthen your spine, but relax your shoulders and your breathing.

Visualise a deep, low muscular belt under your hands. Gently draw your front hand towards your back hand, as though lightly drawing your lower abdomen towards your spine or tightening the belt just one notch.

Although the setting action is sometimes called abdominal bracing, it should feel subtle and light. If you cheat by sucking in your waist or by holding your breath the action becomes ineffective, as you will be recruiting outer muscles without reaching the deep stabilising muscles.

A pelvic floor contraction is another way to initiate core stabilisation. The pelvic floor, deep abdominal and back muscles all work together as a team, so contracting one activates the others.

The pelvic floor is the muscular base of the pelvis, running from the pubic bone to the tailbone. To contract your pelvic floor tighten the muscles as though you are avoiding passing wind or 'holding on' when you need to empty your bladder. Hold this for 5 counts and aim to gradually increase the hold time for stronger endurance.

Abdominal setting and pelvic floor contractions are both great approaches to activating core control. Either action will effectively turn on the 'foundation' muscles to provide deep support.

As you develop strength and an improved awareness of core control you will be able to perform both actions simultaneously. This is the ideal core stabilising method. Sitting tall, draw your naval towards your spine and raise your pelvic floor away from the ball. Hold this gentle bracing while breathing normally.

Adding movement and strength training on the ball further challenges and strengthens core control.

all about balls

There are numerous exercise balls on the market. They vary in colour, size, cost and, most importantly, quality.

Be sure to choose one that is 'anti-burst' or 'burst-resistant'. Not only are these much safer but also they are stronger and more likely to maintain their shape and size. Cheaper balls are often more shiny and slippery, making them less safe in certain positions.

When you are sitting on your exercise ball, your knees and hips should be at 90 degrees, or slightly higher. Using a ball that is too small compromises your seated posture. A larger one makes other exercises too awkward.

The amount you inflate your ball affects its size and the level of challenge it provides. As a general guide, the ball should be firm, with a little give. A slightly firmer ball is more challenging to stabilise and balance, though rock-hard may be uncomfortable.

You can inflate your ball with anything that would blow up an inflatable mattress. A hand or foot-pump will do, as will reverse-cycle vacuums or compressors.

When you first inflate your ball, pump it up until it feels firm but not tight like a drum. It will look smaller than you might expect, but you'll find it 'relaxes' in a day or two, at which time you can top it up to your desired size or firmness.

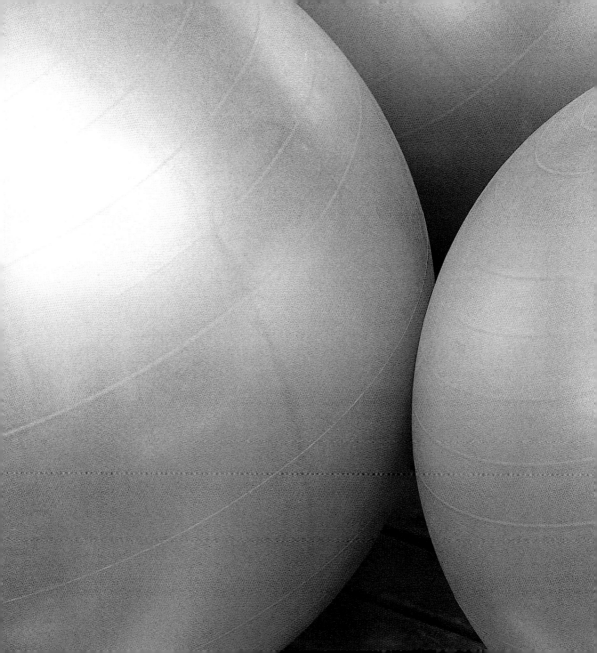

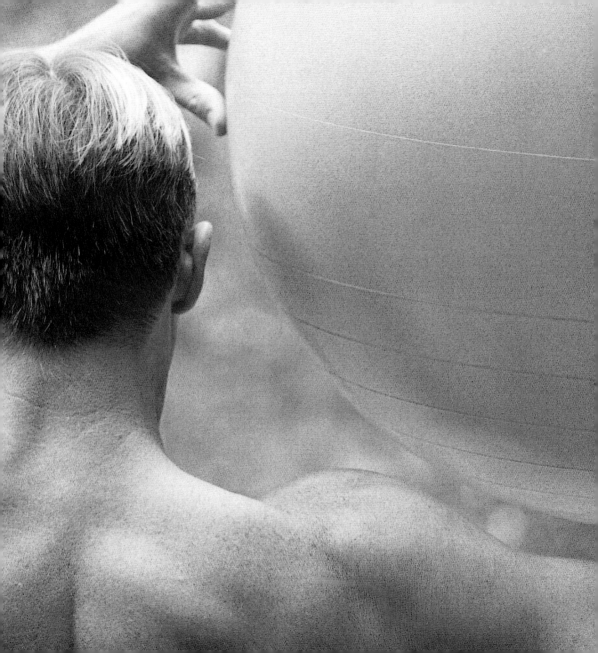

warming-up on the ball

To prepare for your workout, warm up with these mobility options on the ball.

Alternatively, do 10 to 30 minutes of cardiovascular exercise before beginning your ball workout.

Perform the following warm-up moves slowly and smoothly.

Make sure you practise setting your abs (page 26) before beginning your training on the ball.

reach and squat

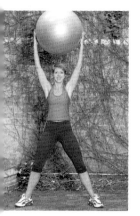 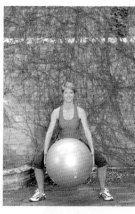

- Stand tall with your feet wide, holding the ball above your head.
- Bend your knees and lower the ball towards the floor, keeping your back straight and upright.
- Straighten your knees and reach up again.
- Repeat x 5

circles

- Starting at the top, take the ball in a big sweeping circle, down towards the floor, back up the other side to the top, then returning the other way.
- Keep your back straight.
- Repeat x 2 each side

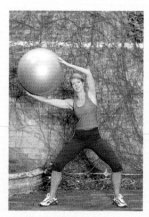 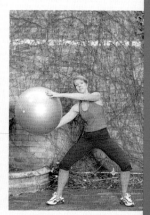

side lunges

- Place the ball on the floor in front of you.
- Feet wide, knees bent, back straight and upright.
- Bending one knee then the other, lunge from side to side and roll the ball side to side.
- Reach across your body, taking your hand towards your opposite knee.

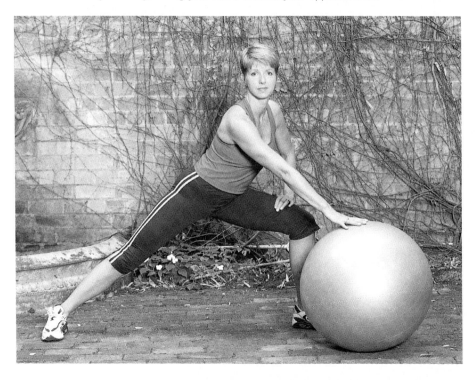

hip circles

- Sit tall on the ball.
- Circle your hips slowly, three times to the right.
- Repeat to the left.

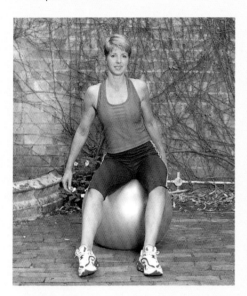 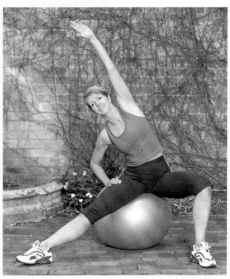

side reaches

- Sit forward on the ball with your hands on your thighs and your back straight.
- Roll the ball to your right, bending your right knee and reaching your right hand to the ceiling.
- Repeat to the left and then to each side again.

back roll

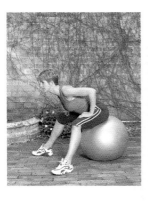 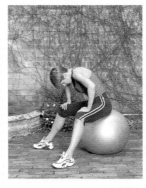

- Sitting forward on the ball with your hands on your thighs and a straight back.
- Lean forward from your hips and then roll slowly back up.
- Start rolling up vertebra by vertebra from the lower back and finish the movement by rolling your shoulder blades back and down.

back and chest stretch

- Sit tall on the ball with your feet hip-width apart.
- Bring your arms forward at chest height.
- Clasp your hands together and gently push forward to round your upper back.
- At the same time, roll the ball forward to round your lower back.
- Reverse this by taking your arms behind you as you roll the ball back and gently arch your spine.

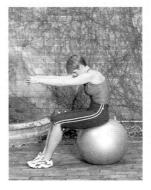 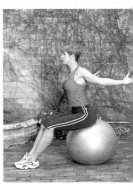

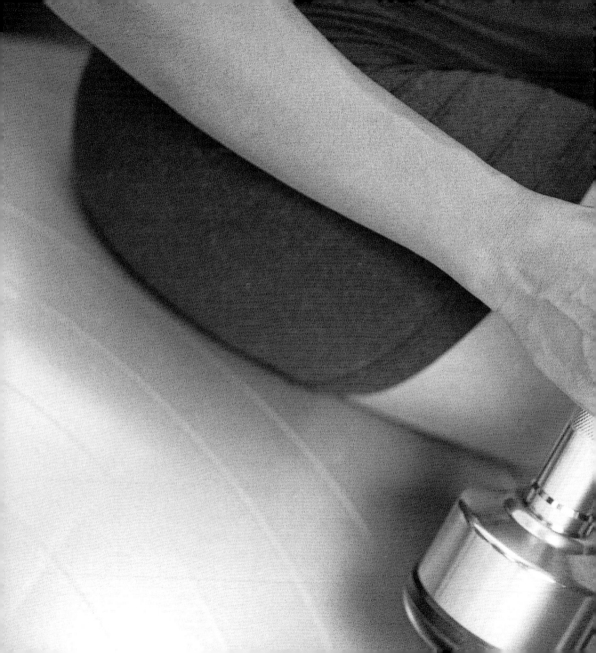

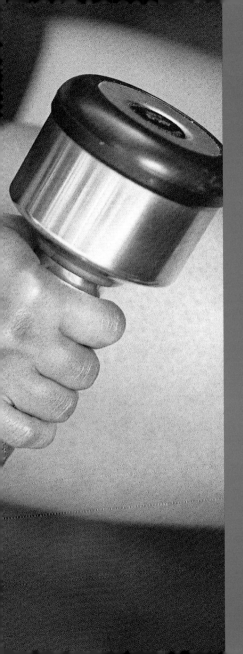

Sitting on the ball to perform upper body strengthening increases the intensity and challenge of your workout, allowing you to train outer muscles for definition and deep muscles for stability.

Sitting tall on an unstable base stimulates activity in the deep abdominal and back muscles. Applying weight training in this position further tests your ability to hold your spine straight and strong, so you simultaneously strengthen your core while toning your upper body.

You can increase the recruitment of the deep spinal stabilisers by altering your base of support. You can do this by bringing your feet together or by adding leg movements, such as taking one foot off the ground.

Anything you do standing or sitting can be done seated on the ball for fresh challenge.

Your rewards are fabulous posture, deep stability and a defined upper body.

seated on the ball

sitting on the ball

getting started

Familiarise yourself with the unstable base provided by the ball and start to improve your core stability by simply sitting on it. It's harder than you think!

Starting position
- Sit on top or slightly forward on the ball to maintain your natural lumbar curve. Place your feet out from the base of the ball, under your knees and hip-width apart.
- Lengthen your spine and set your abdominals to sit tall.

Action
Basic sit
- Maintain a tall, stable seated position on the ball.

Decrease the challenge
- If you're feeling a little unsteady at first, place the ball against the wall until you get the feel of sitting on an unstable base.

Increase the challenge
- A narrower base of support, ie having your feet closer together, creates less stability so the spinal stabilising muscles work harder.
- Add simple arm movements.
- Try taking one foot off the ground.

TRAINER TIPS

BE SURE TO SET YOUR ABDOMINALS AND KEEP YOUR SPINE LENGTHENED.

DO NOT DROP OR SLOUCH.

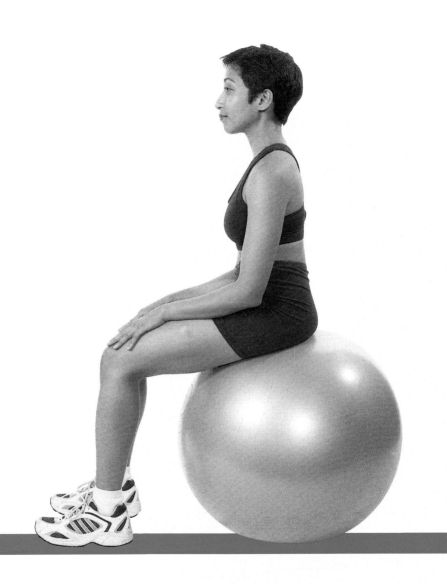

seated leg raise

strengthen your core to support your spine

Starting position
- Sit tall on the ball.
- Relax your arms by your sides.
- Draw your shoulder blades back and down.
- Keep your feet no further than hip-width apart and under your knees.

Action

Leg raise
- Set your abdominals to keep your back tall and in a neutral lumbar curve.
- Raise one heel slowly to knee height, straightening the knee.
- Lower then repeat on the other side.
- 10 reps each side

Decrease the challenge
- Initially rest your fingers on the side of the ball to assist your balance.
- Raise just the heel off the floor.

Increase the challenge
- Extend your arms sideways at shoulder height.
- Hold each leg up for 5 slow counts (or longer).

TRAINER TIPS

KEEP YOUR BACK, PELVIS AND THE BALL STILL.

IT IS TEMPTING TO USE THE THIGH MUSCLE ON THE OTHER LEG TO CONTROL THE BALL, SO SET YOUR ABDOMINALS AND RELAX THE THIGH TO AVOID CHEATING.

STRETCH
HIP CIRCLES PAGE 159

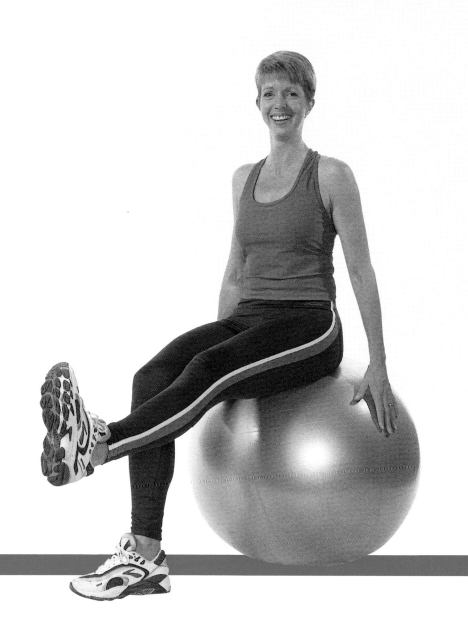

lateral arm raise

shapely shoulders

Starting position
- Use your level 2 weights.
- Sit on the ball holding a weight in each hand.
- Place your elbows by your sides and bend them to 90 degrees.

Action
Side raise
- Raise your arms sideways until your forearms are horizontal and level with your shoulders.
- Lower back down, bringing your elbows back to your sides.
- 15 reps x 2

Decrease the challenge
- Start with your level 1 weights (or no weights) and do 1 set of 15.
- Gradually build up to 2 sets of 15 and then increase your weights when you are ready.

Increase the challenge
- Increase to 20 reps x 2
- Do lateral raises with one leg off the ground, keeping your back straight and the ball still. Change legs to perform the second set. Keep your posture upright.

Go harder
- Do unilateral raises, ie one arm at a time, repeating 15 reps on each arm, to further challenge stabilisation. Do not lean on the other arm.
- Combine a single-arm lateral raise with a leg raise for a greater challenge.
- Raise the same leg as the working arm for your toughest option.

TRAINER TIPS

AS YOU RAISE YOUR ARMS DRAW YOUR SHOULDER BLADES DOWNWARDS.

YOUR HANDS AND WEIGHTS GO NO HIGHER THAN YOUR ELBOWS.

AVOID RAISING YOUR SHOULDERS AND TENSING MUSCLES IN THE NECK.

STRETCH

NECK AND SHOULDERS STRETCH PAGE 160

TAKE CARE

IF YOU FEEL DISCOMFORT IN THE NECK OR SHOULDERS, CHECK YOUR TECHNIQUE OR OMIT THIS EXERCISE.

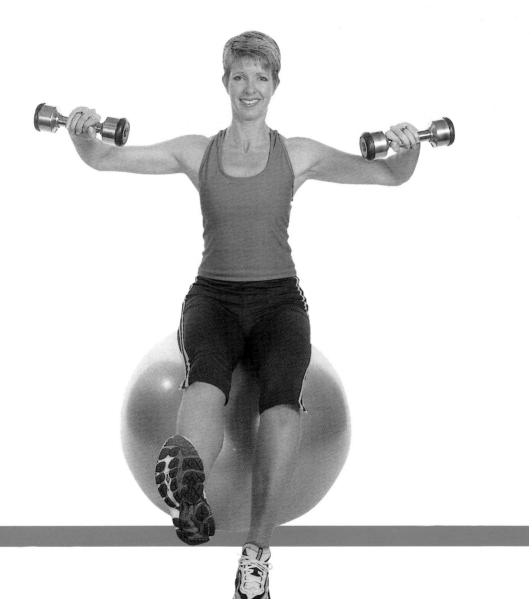

shoulder press

strong defined shoulders for function and form

Starting position
- Use your level 2 weights.
- Sit tall and set your abdominals.
- Hold your weights beside your shoulders, ready to press to the ceiling.

Action
Press up and pull down
- Press the weights upwards and towards each other.
- Lower them slowly bringing your elbows slightly backwards and drawing your shoulder blades together to recruit your upper back muscles.
- 15 reps x 3

Decrease the challenge
- Start with your level 1 weights and gradually build up.

Increase the challenge
- Increase weights, number of reps or sets.
- Add an alternate leg raise to further train spinal stabilisers.

TRAINER TIPS

YOUR HANDS SHOULD TRAVEL SLIGHTLY FORWARDS AS THEY GO UP AND SLIGHTLY BACKWARDS AS THEY COME DOWN SO THE MOVEMENT IS ANGLED GENTLY FORWARD.

RELAX YOUR NECK AND AVOID HITCHING YOUR SHOULDERS TOWARDS YOUR EARS AS THIS CAN CAUSE UNNECESSARY TENSION IN YOUR NECK.

STRETCH

NECK AND SHOULDERS
STRETCH PAGE 160

TAKE CARE

AVOID THIS EXERCISE IF YOU HAVE ANY NECK OR SHOULDER DISCOMFORT.

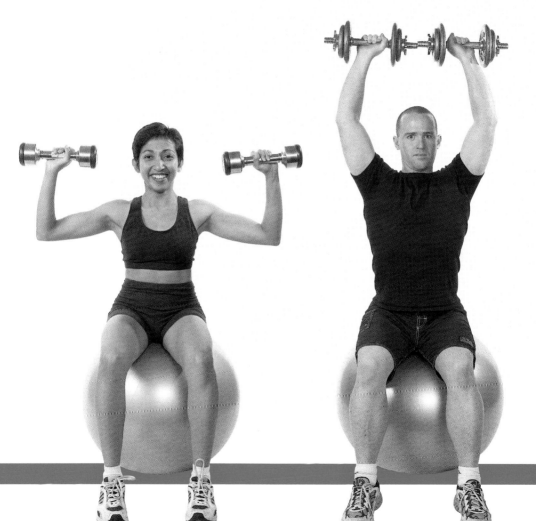

seated row

define your back and shoulders

Starting position

- Use your level 2 weights.
- Sit tall, holding a weight in each hand, palms facing upwards.
- Place your elbows by your sides, bent to 90 degrees.
- Draw your shoulder blades back and down.

Action

Reach forward and pull back

- Reach forward, taking the weights to your knees.
- Pull your elbows backwards and your hands towards your hips.
- 15 reps x 2

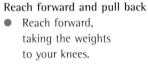

TRAINER TIPS

CONSCIOUSLY PULL YOUR SHOULDERS BACK AND DOWN AS YOU BRING YOUR ARMS BACKWARDS TO EMPHASISE THE IMPORTANT UPPER BACK COMPONENT OF THIS EXERCISE.

STRETCH

BACK AND CHEST
STRETCH PAGE 35

Decrease the challenge
● Use your level 1 weights while you fine-tune your technique and form.

Increase the challenge
● Perform a third set.

Go harder
● Add an alternating leg raise to each row to further test your ability to stabilise.

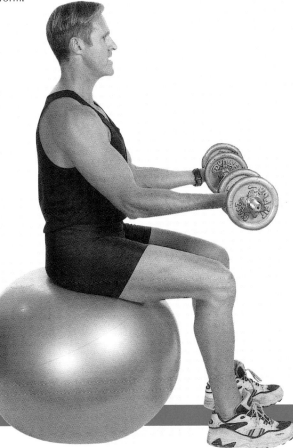

seated triceps press

show off firm upper arms

Starting position
- Use one of your level 3 weights.
- Hold it in both hands, behind your head.
- Keep your elbows close to your forehead.

Action
Press to the sky
- Press the weight towards the ceiling, straightening your elbows.
- Bend your elbows to lower the weight slowly back down behind your head.
- 15 reps x 2

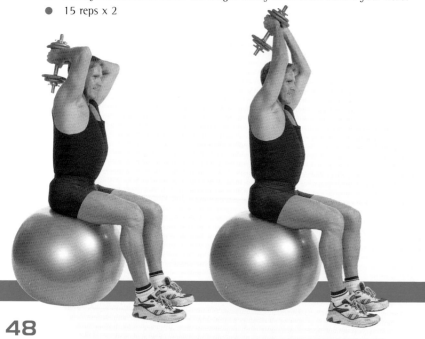

TRAINER TIPS

VISUALISE PUSHING
THE WEIGHT UPWARDS,
NOT FORWARDS.

KEEP YOUR ELBOWS TUCKED
IN, CLOSE TO YOUR FOREHEAD.

STRETCH

TRICEPS STRETCH PAGE 160

TAKE CARE

AVOID THIS EXERCISE IF YOU
HAVE ANY NECK, ELBOW OR
SHOULDER DISCOMFORT.

Decrease the challenge
● Use your level 1 or 2 weights.
● You may prefer to do triceps press back, (page 104).

Increase the challenge
● Increase the weight or perform a third set.
● Raise one leg at a time straightening your knee as you raise the weight.

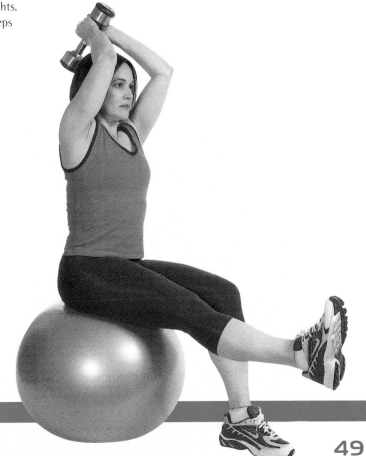

49

triceps dip

the ultimate challenge for triceps strength and shoulder stability

This is an advanced exercise requiring strict form and technique. It is only suitable for people who are confident performing tricep dips. You may feel this exercise more in the upper back, in the muscles that stabilise the shoulder girdle, and less in the triceps compared to a traditional triceps dip.

Starting position
- Sit tall on the ball.
- Place your hands beside your hips, fingers pointing forwards.
- Step forward with each foot to take your bottom just off the ball.
- Set your abdominals and straighten your spine.
- Your weight is in the heels of your hands on the ball, and the heels of your feet on the floor.

Action
Bend elbows to dip
- Bend your elbows, lowering your body downwards.
- 10 reps x 2

Decrease the challenge
- Build up your confidence by doing dips on a stable base such as a bench before trying them on the exercise ball.
- Rest the ball against a wall to make the dip more stable.
- Do the seated triceps press (page 48) as an alternative.

Increase the challenge
- Place your feet further out from the ball.

TRAINER TIPS
KEEP YOUR BACK STRAIGHT AND YOUR HIPS DIRECTLY UNDER YOUR SHOULDERS.

YOUR BOTTOM SHOULD ALMOST SLIDE DOWN THE FRONT OF THE BALL (KEEP IT CLOSE).

STRETCH
TRICEPS STRETCH PAGE 160

TAKE CARE
THIS EXERCISE IS UNSAFE ON A SLIPPERY SURFACE. BE SURE YOUR FLOOR IS NON-SLIP

THIS EXERCISE IS INAPPROPRIATE IF YOU HAVE A WRIST, SHOULDER OR NECK PROBLEM OR ARE NEW TO EXERCISE BALL OR STRENGTH TRAINING.

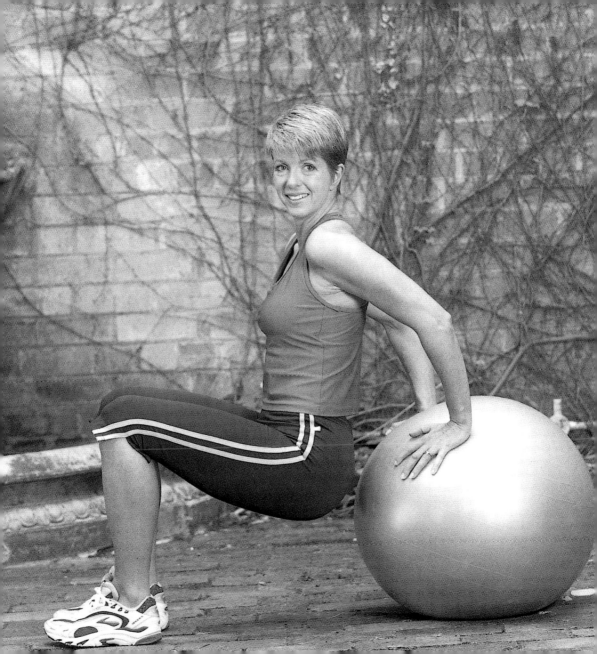

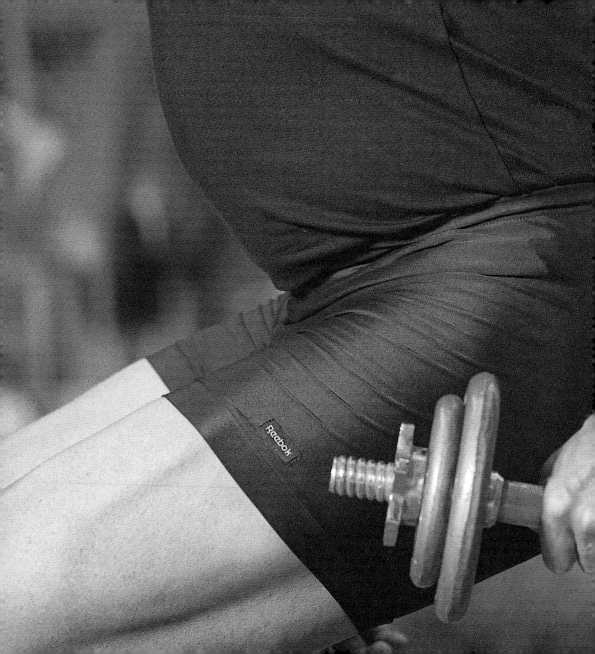

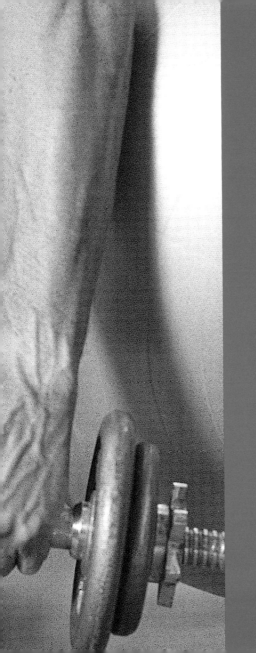

The exercise ball and a wall make a great team, providing excellent exercise variety.

The wall is sometimes used to support the ball, which lessens instability and makes wall exercises easier for the beginner. Resting the ball against the wall can be useful, for example, for getting used to sitting on the ball when you first start.

In the following exercises, the ball and wall combination provide a fresh approach to traditional exercises such as push-ups, squats and lunges. In all cases, the exercises require the use of extra stabilising musculature to maintain posture, leading to heightened benefits and a whole new challenge.

standing with the ball

wall squat

long, lean legs plus power for lifting

Starting position

- Stand with your back to the wall and feet hip-width apart.
- Place the ball between your lower back and the wall.
- Lower yourself to a seated squat position, ie thighs are horizontal.
- Set your abdominals and keep your back straight.
- Move your feet away from the wall until you can see your toes just beyond your knees.

Action

Stand and sit

- Slowly stand up, then sit back down in the squat position.
- 20 reps x 2

Decrease the challenge

- Try a semi-squat first by not sitting so low.
- Decrease the number of reps or do one set only.

Increase the challenge

- Hold weights by your side to further load the quadriceps. Start with the lightest and progress to the heaviest as your strength increases.
- Try to do a single-leg squat by placing your second foot lightly on the floor for balance or off the ground for more difficulty. Keep your back straight and don't lean sideways. 20 reps each side

TRAINER TIPS

TO TAKE THE STRESS OFF YOUR KNEES, KEEP YOUR BODY WEIGHT BACK IN YOUR HEELS AND CHECK YOU CAN ALWAYS SEE YOUR TOES.

KEEP YOUR BACK STRAIGHT AND PARALLEL TO THE WALL, IE DON'T LEAN FORWARD OR BACK.

SET YOUR ABDOMINALS THROUGHOUT.

STRETCH

QUADS STRETCH PAGE 152

TAKE CARE

DISCONTINUE IF YOU FEEL DISCOMFORT IN YOUR KNEES.

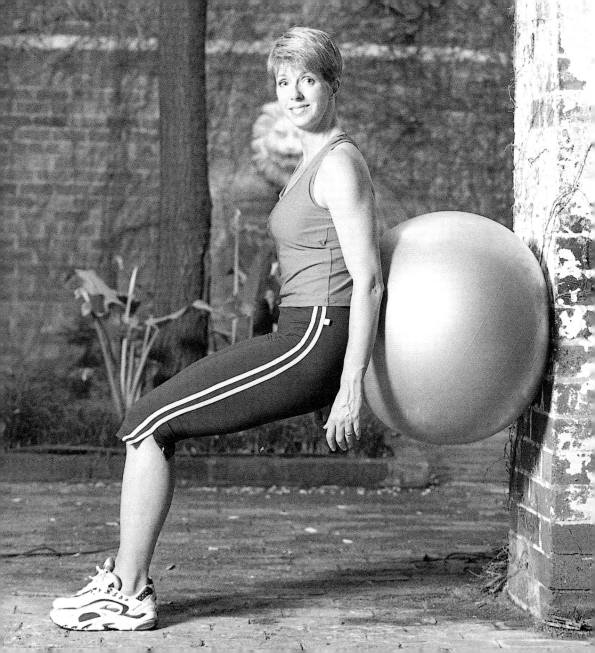

wall squat
with bicep curl
arms and legs take shape together

Starting position
- Use your level 2 weights.
- Hold the weights in your hands while you position the ball behind your back.
- Lower yourself to a seated squat position, ie thighs are horizontal.
- Your arms are straight and by your sides.

Action
Stand and sit with bicep curl
- Stand up slowly and bend your elbows to raise the weights towards your shoulders.
- Now sit down again (squat) as you lower the weights and straighten your elbows.
- 15 reps x 3

Decrease the challenge
- Use your level 1 weights.
- 15 reps x 2

Increase the challenge
- Use your level 3 weights.
- Perform a single-leg squat and single-arm bicep curl. Shift your weight almost completely onto one foot, using the other foot for balance only. Set your abdominals and do not lean sideways.

Go harder
- Perform other upper-body exercises in conjunction with the wall squat such as the lateral raise (page 42) or shoulder press (page 44).

TRAINER TIPS

KEEP YOUR ELBOWS TUCKED IN AND BACK AGAINST THE BALL.

ENSURE YOU FULLY BEND AND STRAIGHTEN YOUR ELBOWS TO TAKE YOUR ARMS THROUGH THE FULL RANGE OF MOVEMENT.

STRETCH

QUADS STRETCH PAGE 152
PECS STRETCH PAGE 147

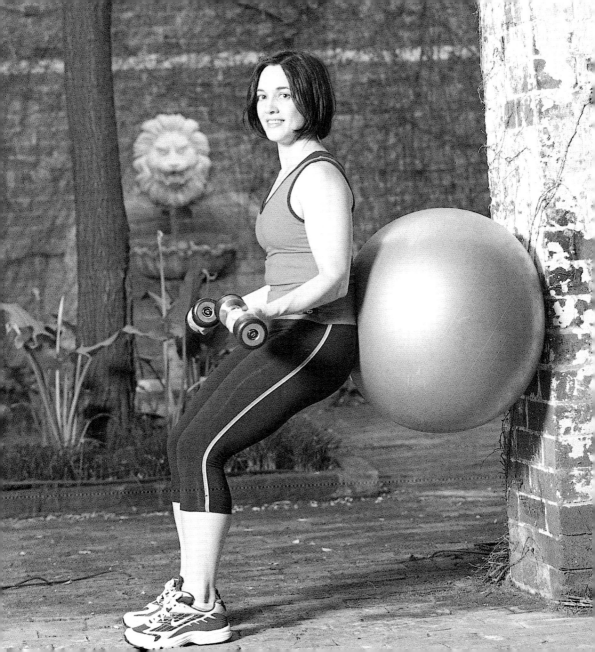

wall lunge

sensational thighs and toned butt

Starting position

- Position the ball between your lower back and the wall.
- Place one foot as far forward as possible, and the other back close to the wall with your heel off the ground.
- Keeping your back straight, lean slightly forward so that your tailbone is touching the ball.
- Set your abdominals.

Action

Lunge and stand

- Bending both knees, lower yourself down slowly until your front knee is bent to approximately 90 degrees.
- Now stand back up.
- 15 reps x 2

Decrease the challenge

- If you are just starting out or feel any discomfort in the knees, do not lunge as deeply or go as low into the squat initially.

Increase the challenge

- Hold your level 2 or 3 weights by your side to further load the quadriceps.

TRAINER TIPS

KEEP YOUR BACK STRAIGHT BUT SLIGHTLY INCLINED FORWARD, IE WITH YOUR CHEST UP.

KEEP THE WEIGHT IN YOUR FRONT HEEL, AND THE BALL OF YOUR BACK FOOT.

DEEPER LUNGES ARE MORE INTENSE, SO BEND LOWER FOR A HARDER WORKOUT.

LEAN BACK INTO THE BALL TO CHANGE LEGS.

STRETCH

QUADS STRETCH PAGE 152

TAKE CARE

MODIFY OR OMIT THIS EXERCISE IF YOU HAVE ANY KNEE DISCOMFORT.

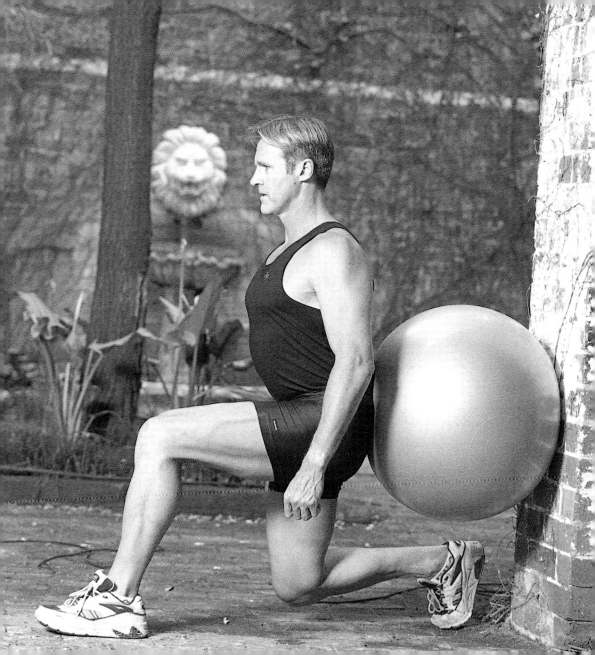

lunge with upright row

strongly defined above and below

Starting position
- Use your level 2 weights.
- Position the exercise ball between your tailbone and the wall.
- Place one foot foward in lunge position.
- Hold the weights either side of your front knee.

Action
Lunge and straighten with weights
- Lunge up and down, raising the weights to chest height as you lunge downwards and lowering them towards the floor as you stand back up.
- 15 reps x 2

Decrease the challenge
- Stick to the wall lunge exercise (page 58) then progress to the lunge with upright row when you are ready.

Increase the challenge
- Use your level 3 weights.
- Hold the lunge position while you perform 15 upright rows. Change legs and repeat.

TRAINER TIPS

YOUR ELBOWS SHOULD FINISH SLIGHTLY HIGHER THAN YOUR WEIGHTS.

KEEP YOUR WRISTS STRONG.

KEEP YOUR SHOULDER BLADES BACK AND DOWN.

STRETCH

QUADS STRETCH PAGE 152
NECK AND SHOULDER STRETCH PAGE 160

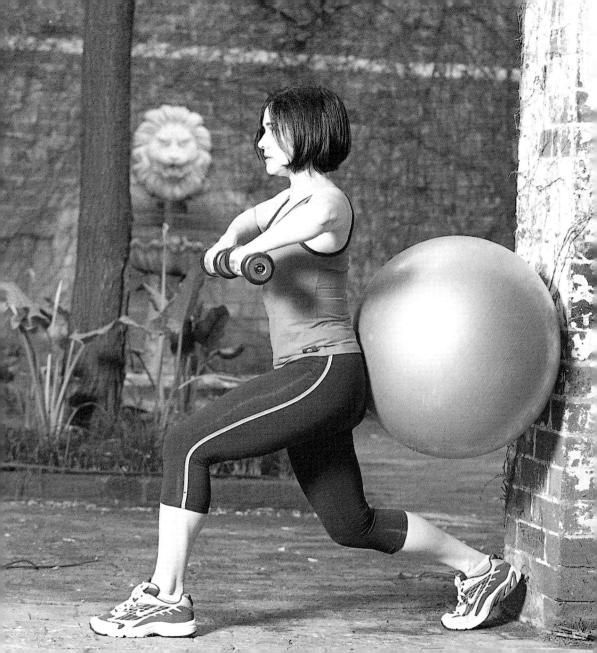

wall push-up

more strength, less stress

Strengthens your chest and arms with less stress on your lower back than a regular push-up and with extra emphasis on upper back and shoulder stability.

Starting position
- Stand holding the ball at chest height between you and the wall.
- Place your hands on the ball at shoulder height.
- Holding the ball against the wall, step back.
- Head, neck, spine and pelvis in a straight line.

Action
Push-up towards the wall
- Move your chest towards the wall, bending your elbows outwards.
- Press back away from the wall to straighten your arms.
- 15 reps x 2

Decrease the challenge
- Move closer to the wall to make the exercise less intense or to lighten the load on your shoulders.

Increase the challenge
- Walk your feet further out from the wall to increase intensity.
- Lift one foot off the floor to challenge your deeper muscles. Be sure to keep your pelvis square to the wall.

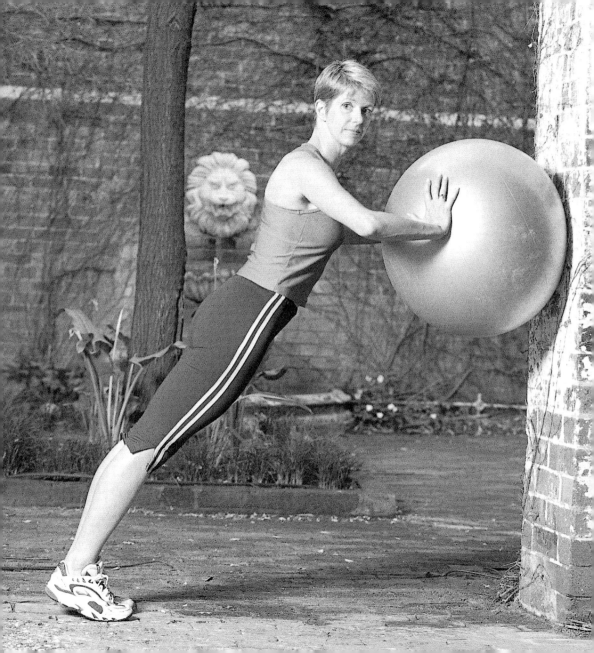

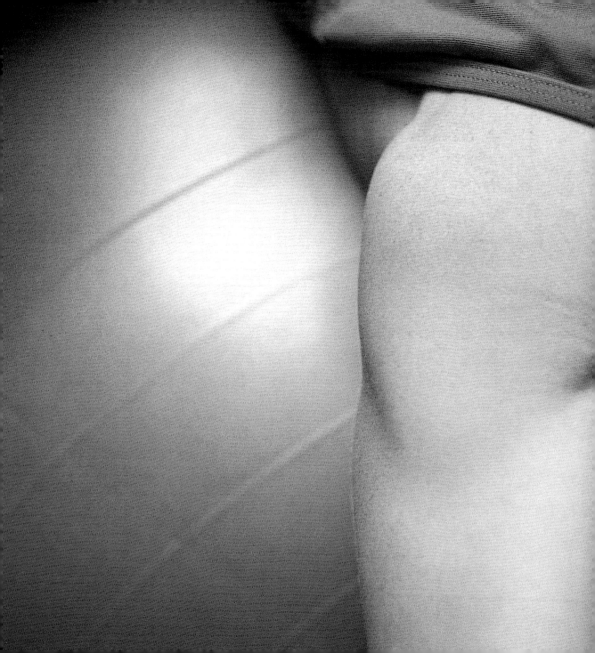

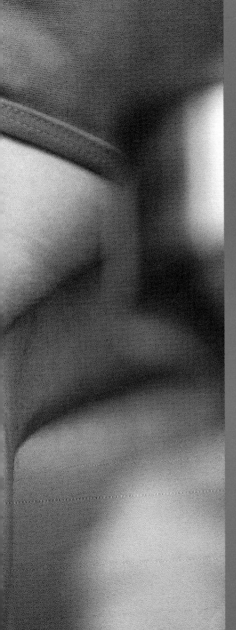

When you are in the supine position, you lie face up on the exercise ball. In this position your head, neck and shoulders are well supported, but your back and pelvis are not. This means you recruit many deep muscles to stabilise your torso and hold your pelvis and hips up, particularly your gluteals and your spinal stabilisers.

Supine on the ball provides a great alternative to the bench for exercises such as chest press and lat pullover. Using an unstable base and having an unsupported pelvis brings several other important muscles into the action, such as the deep abdominals and gluteals, as well as the target muscle group in the upper body. Once again, strength and core stability unite to create a powerful and efficient mode of exercise.

Not only do the supine exercises combine core conditioning with outer strength but they are also excellent butt-busters!

Practise rolling in and out of supine to start with and familiarise yourself with the technique points of the position so you can perform the other supine exercises correctly.

supine on the ball

rolling in and out of supine

getting started

In order to perform the supine exercises, you need to be able to roll in and out of the position with ease.

Starting position
● Sit on the ball with your hands by your sides.

Action
Roll in and out of supine
● To move into the supine position, walk your feet out, rolling your hips down and lying back on the ball as you do so. Stop when your shoulder blades are on the ball.
● Lower your head to the ball and raise your hips.
● Hold for 5 slow counts.
● To move out of the supine position, drop your hips and raise your head off the ball.
● Press your lower back into the ball and slowly walk back up to the sitting position.
● Repeat x 3

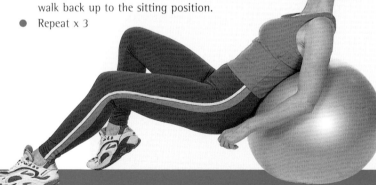

TRAINER TIPS
KEEP YOUR NECK IN LINE WITH YOUR SPINE.

IF YOUR CHIN IS ON YOUR CHEST AS IN THE SMALL PHOTO OPPOSITE, WALK BACK A LITTLE.

IF YOUR HEAD IS HANGING BACK OVER THE BALL, WALK FURTHER FORWARD.

KEEP YOUR HIPS UP LEVEL WITH YOUR SPINE AND SET YOUR ABDOMINALS TO SUPPORT AND STABILISE YOUR BACK.

PRESS THROUGH YOUR HEELS AND CONTRACT YOUR GLUTEALS TO KEEP YOUR HIPS UP

STRETCH
BACK AND BUTT STRETCH PAGE 158

Decrease the challenge

● Roll into the position and out again without holding.
● Repeat x 3

Increase the challenge

● Bring your feet together to further strengthen your stabilisers.

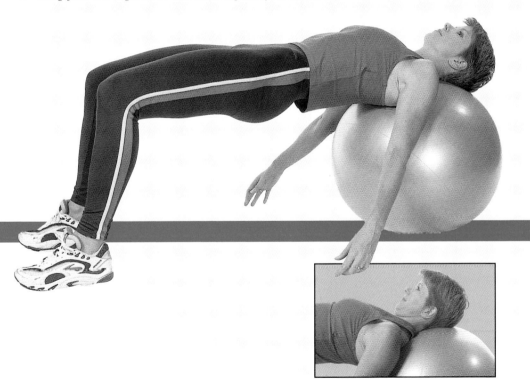

ball bridges

linking backs and butts

Starting position

- Supine on the ball with head and shoulders supported.
- Place your hands wherever is comfortable—under your head, resting on your hips or down by your side.
- Keep your feet hip-width apart or closer.
- Head, neck, spine and pelvis horizontal and in line.

Action

Lower and raise hips

- Set your abdominals and lower your butt towards the floor.
- Press through your heels and contract your gluteals to raise your hips back up to the horizontal position.
- 15 reps x 3

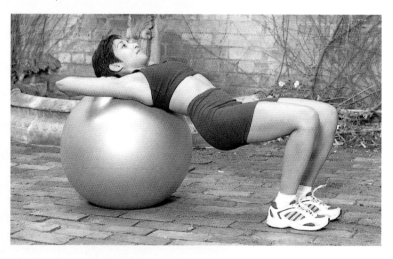

TRAINER TIPS

KEEP THE WEIGHT IN YOUR HEELS. YOU SHOULD BE ABLE TO WRIGGLE YOUR TOES.

STRONGLY SET YOUR ABDOMINALS – IT'S IMPORTANT TO SUPPORT YOUR BACK IN THIS EXERCISE.

STRETCH

BACK ROLL PAGE 35

TAKE CARE

IF YOU FEEL DISCOMFORT IN THE LOWER BACK CHECK THAT YOU ARE SETTING YOUR ABDOMINALS. IF THE DISCOMFORT PERSISTS DISCONTINUE THE EXERCISE.

Decrease the challenge
- Start with rolling in and out of supine (page 66) or try bridging on the floor instead of the ball.

Increase the challenge
- Place your feet close and squeeze your knees together at the top of each raise.
- Keeping your heels on the ground, lift your toes off the floor.

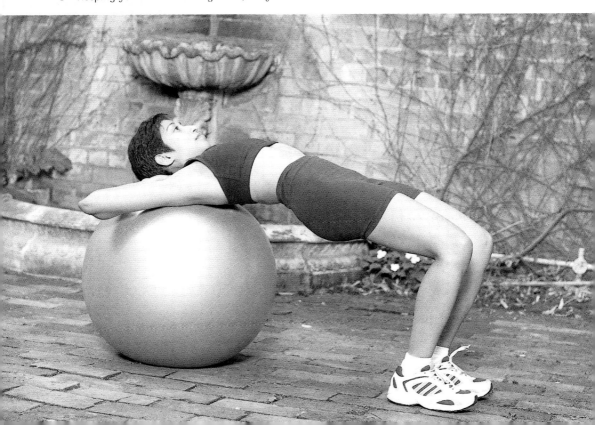

supine stability

shifting weight for great core control

Starting position
- Supine on the ball.
- Rest hands on hips, under head or arms down at sides.

Action
Glide from side to side
- Slowly shift your weight across to one foot, then to the other, keeping both feet on the ground.
- Keep your pelvis horizontal.
- 10 reps, each side

Decrease the challenge
- Simply raise one heel then the other off the ground.

Increase the challenge
- Shift your weight carefully to one foot, then raise the other leg to extend the knee. Hold for 5 slow counts before changing legs.
- Gradually increase the time you hold each side.

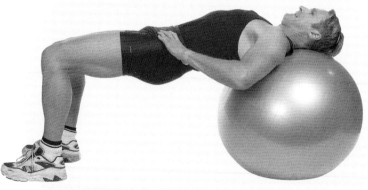

TRAINER TIPS

USE YOUR GLUTEALS TO KEEP YOUR PELVIS SQUARE AND AVOID DROPPING EITHER HIP.

SET YOUR ABDOMINALS TO MAINTAIN SPINAL SUPPORT AND CONTROL.

KEEP THE OTHER FOOT LIGHTLY ON THE GROUND FOR BALANCE UNTIL YOU HAVE HAD CONSIDERABLE PRACTICE AT THIS EXERCISE.

STRETCH
BACK AND BUTT
STRETCH PAGE 158

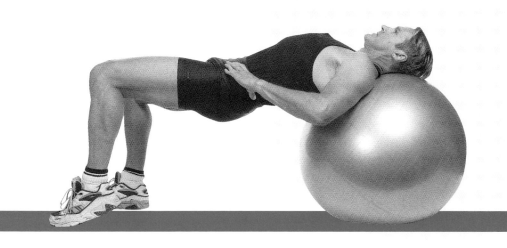

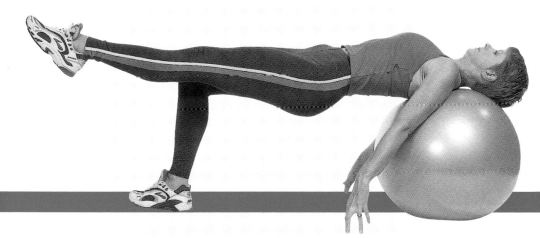

71

chest press

pecs of perfection

Starting position
- Use your level 3 weights.
- Hold a weight in each hand and walk down into the supine position, lowering your elbows to the ball to guide the way.
- Keep your feet hip-width apart.
- Extend your arms towards the ceiling, with your weights directly above your chest.

Action
Lower and press
- Bend your elbows to lower the weights down and outwards.
- Slowly press back up.
- 15 reps x 3

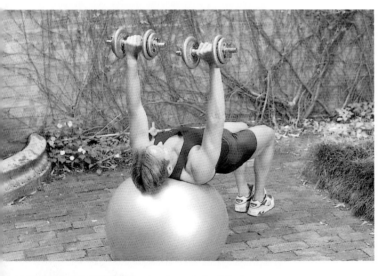

TRAINER TIPS
KEEP YOUR NECK IN NEUTRAL POSITION, IN LINE WITH YOUR SPINE.

ALLOW YOUR ELBOWS TO ARC OUTWARDS AND DOWN TO SHOULDER LEVEL OR A LITTLE LOWER. THE BALL WILL HELP TO CONTROL THIS RANGE OF MOVEMENT.

SET YOUR ABDOMINALS TO SUPPORT YOUR BACK.

KEEP THE WEIGHT IN YOUR HEELS AND YOUR HIPS RAISED.

STRETCH
PECS STRETCH PAGE 147

Decrease the challenge
- Initially try this exercise with your level 2 weights then build up.
- Lower your hips after each set to rest the gluteals and back muscles.

Increase the challenge
- Increase the number of reps or your weights.
- Move your feet closer together.
- Work one arm at a time to further challenge pelvic and spinal stability.

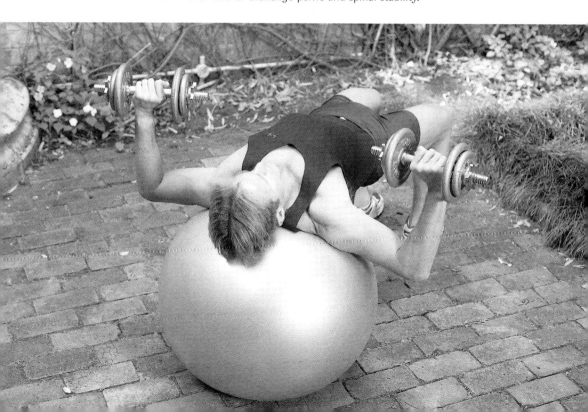

flys

tougher than your trad fly

Starting position
- Use your level 2 weights.
- Supine on the ball.
- Extend your arms straight up towards the ceiling, holding your weights above the chest.
- Palms face each other and elbows are almost straight.

Action
Open and close
- Slowly lower your arms out sideways, keeping elbows slightly bent.
- Contract your chest muscles and raise the weights back towards each other.
- 15 reps x 2

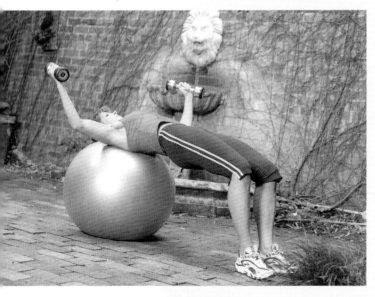

TRAINER TIPS

FLYS ARE A LONGER LEVER EXERCISE SO SHOULD ALWAYS BE PERFORMED SLOWLY, ESPECIALLY WHEN USING HEAVIER WEIGHTS.

SET YOUR ABDOMINALS TO SUPPORT YOUR BACK.

TIGHTEN YOUR GLUTEALS TO STABILISE YOUR PELVIS.

AVOID HYPEREXTENSION (ARCHING YOUR SPINE).

STRETCH
PECS STRETCH PAGE 147

Decrease the challenge
● To familiarise yourself with the action, start with your level 1 weights, ensuring correct positioning and control.

Increase the challenge
● Bring your feet closer together to increase the workload for the pelvic and lumbar stabilisers.
● Increase weights and number of reps.

Go harder
● Follow the basic action with single-arm flys for extra challenge around the mid-section and pelvis. Lower one weight as for a fly, keeping the other arm directly above your chest. Do not let the ball move sideways, and don't let your hips drop. Build up to 10 reps on each side.

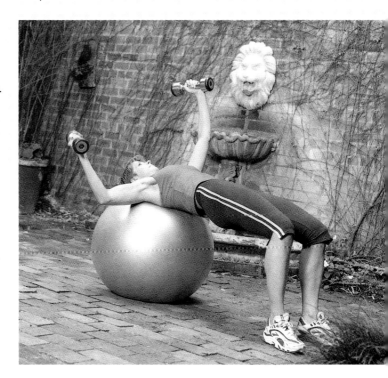

lat pullover

shape and definition for a sculpted back

Latissimus dorsi is the back muscle that is particularly well developed in swimmers, giving them the shape that many of us admire and desire. This muscle also functions as a pelvic stabiliser in conjunction with the gluteals and so it is ideal to train the two together in the supine position.

Starting position
- Hold one of your level 3 weights in both hands and roll into supine.
- Extend your arms towards the ceiling holding the weight above your chest.

Action
Lower and raise
- Keeping your elbows slightly bent, slowly lower the weight.
- Raise your arms back towards the ceiling.
- 15 reps x 2

Decrease the challenge
- Use your level 2 weight.

Increase the challenge
- Increase weights, number of reps or sets.
- Move feet closer together.

TRAINER TIPS
FOCUS ON A SLOW, CONTROLLED MOVEMENT.

KEEP THE ELBOWS SOFT.

STRETCH
LATS STRETCH PAGE 146

TAKE CARE
AVOID HYPEREXTENSION.

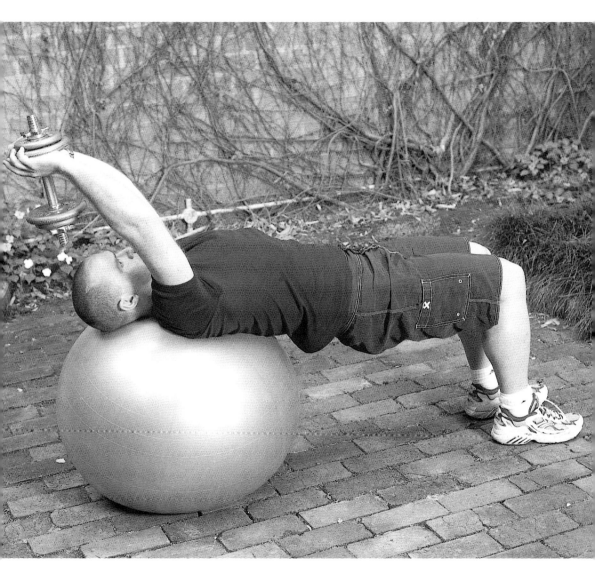

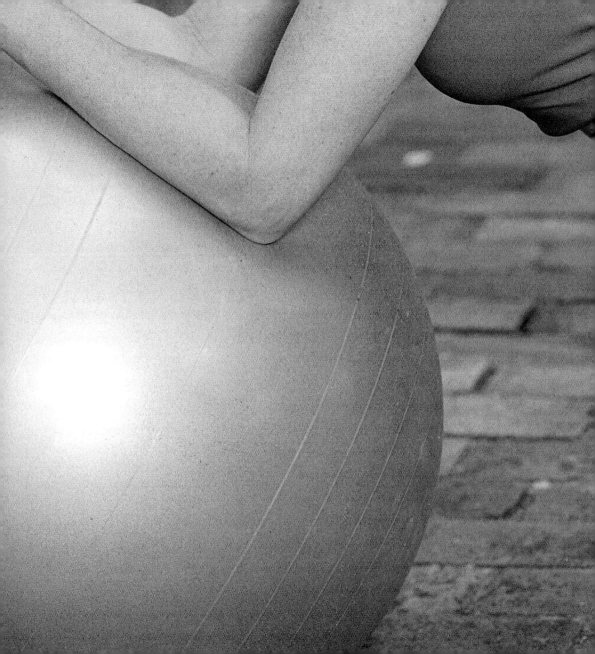

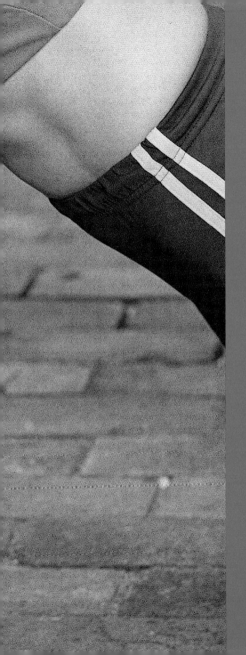

Using the exercise ball for abdominal work brings a whole new meaning to ab training. While outer ab muscles such as rectus abdominus and the external obliques are working, so too are the deeper muscles that support the spine. This means a deeper, more thorough and far more challenging abdominal program.

There's ab training – then there's abs on the ball. Feeling is believing!

abs on the ball

abs on the ball

getting started

Abdominal curls on the ball are tougher than traditional crunches on terra firma. Extra muscle recruitment means added challenge and training benefit.

Abdominal curls that only use the outer muscles such as **rectus abdominus** may harm your back. Not only does this common practice place you at risk but it also decreases your workout value. Always be sure to set your abdominals before and during your abdominal curls and crunches. This recruits the important deep abdominals to stabilise your spine and so works all your abs, from the inside out.

Starting position
- Sit on the ball.
- Take a big step forward with each foot and then roll your lower back down onto the ball.
- Your tailbone, pelvis and lower back must be supported. Make sure your tailbone is touching the ball.
- Place your feet on the floor, directly under your knees or slightly further out from the ball.
- Keep your knees and feet hip-width apart.
- Place your hands behind your head.
- Your neck should be aligned with your spine.

You are now in position to start crunching. Altering the lever length or base of support are both methods of adjusting the intensity of your abdominal training.

TRAINER TIP

DRAWING YOUR NAVAL TOWARDS YOUR SPINE, IE SETTING YOUR ABS DURING EVERY CURL OR OBLIQUE RAISE, WILL MAKE AN INCREDIBLE DIFFERENCE TO THE QUALITY OF YOUR ABDOMINAL TRAINING.

TAKE CARE

ALWAYS KEEP YOUR BUTT IN CONTACT WITH THE BALL.

ALWAYS BRACE YOUR ABS TO SUPPORT YOUR BACK DURING AB CURLS. IF YOU HAVE DISCOMFORT, THEN AB CURLS ON THE FLOOR MAY BE MORE APPROPRIATE. IF YOU HAVE A BACK PROBLEM, STABILISATION EXERCISES ARE MORE SUITABLE THAN CURLS (SEE BACK IN ACTION PROGRAM, PAGE 172)

Decrease the challenge

- Walk a small step forward, allowing your tailbone to rest slightly further down the front of the ball.
- Have your feet hip-width apart.

Increase the challenge

- Walk your body a step further back over the ball, taking your tailbone closer to the top, to lengthen the lever.
- Bring your feet closer together to decrease your base of support and increase deep abdominal involvement.
- Combine the two to make the ab curl even harder. You'll feel the difference.

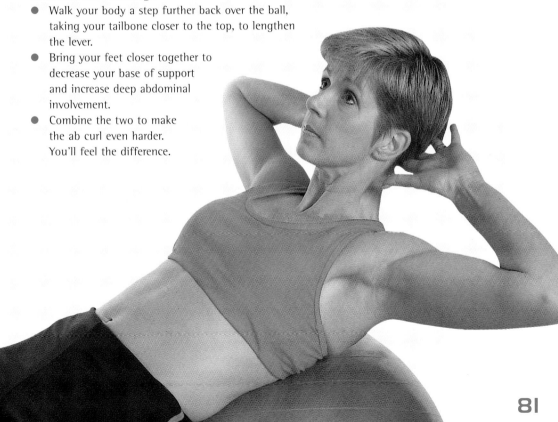

abdominal curls

blitz your abs

Starting position
- Supine with the ball under your lower back and pelvis.
- Place your hands behind your head with elbows back.

Action
Curl fowards
- Set your abdominals, drawing your naval towards the ball.
- Curl your upper body up to a position which is about half-way between lying and sitting.
- Roll slowly back down over the ball.
- 15 reps x 3

Decrease the challenge
- To make the exercise less intense, take a small step forward. Lower your tailbone so it remains in contact with the ball.

Increase the challenge
- Walk a step further back with each foot to take your body slightly further out over the ball. A small step backwards makes a big difference.
- Place feet closer together.
- If you feel confident with ab curls on the ball and have no back problem, try lowering your back a little further over the ball to curl from a slightly extended position.

TRAINER TIPS

DO NOT HOLD YOUR BREATH.

DO NOT PULL ON YOUR HEAD AS IT MAY STRAIN YOUR NECK.

KEEP YOUR CHIN OFF YOUR CHEST AND YOUR NECK IN LINE WITH YOUR SPINE.

AIM TO CREATE A CONCAVE ABDOMEN BY DRAWING YOUR LOWER ABDOMEN INWARDS BEFORE ROLLING UP.

ROLL UP AND DOWN AS THOUGH YOU ARE ROLLING ONE VERTEBRA AT A TIME. IF YOU KEEP YOUR SPINE STRAIGHT, YOU RISK BACK PROBLEMS.

STRETCH
BACK EXTENSION PAGE 162

TAKE CARE

IF YOU ROLL A LONG WAY FORWARD AND ARE HALFWAY DOWN THE FRONT OF THE BALL, YOU MAY SLIP OFF.

IF YOU FEEL YOU NEED TO COME THAT FAR FORWARD IT'S BETTER TO LIE ON THE FLOOR TO PERFORM ABDOMINAL CURLS UNTIL YOU DEVELOP A LITTLE MORE STRENGTH.

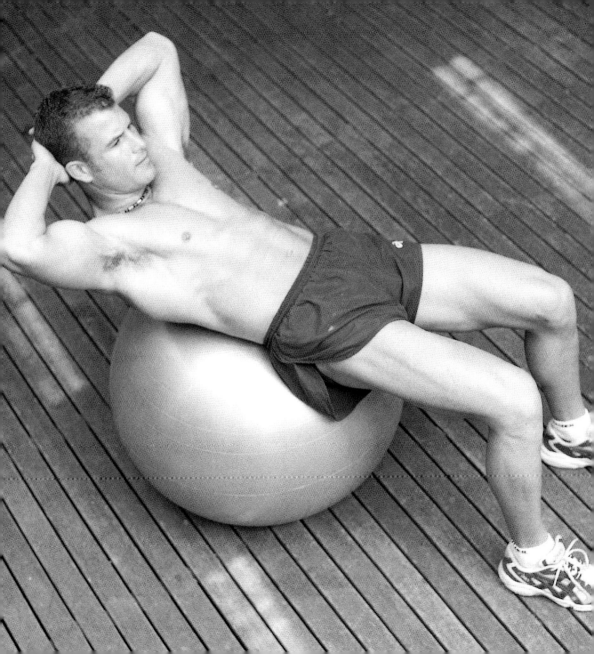

oblique curls

obliques for a sleek torso

Starting position
- Supine with the ball supporting your pelvis and lower back.
- Place your left hand behind your head with the elbow back.
- Extend your right arm up and across your body, reaching your right hand to the ceiling above your left knee.

Action
Reach and raise
- Raise your shoulders and reach your right hand up and across to the left in one smooth movement.
- Roll back down.
- 15 reps each side x 2

Decrease the challenge
- Alternate your oblique curls, one arm then the other.
- Decrease number of reps and sets.

Increase the challenge
- Increase number of reps and sets.
- Hold for 5 slow counts at the top of each oblique curl.
- Feet together.

TRAINER TIPS

SET YOUR ABDOMINALS BEFORE YOU RAISE YOUR SHOULDERS AND HOLD THEM UNTIL YOU RETURN BACK DOWN.

KEEP YOUR ARM EXTENDED, IE ELBOW STRAIGHT.

DO NOT PULL ON YOUR NECK.

DO NOT HOLD YOUR BREATH.

STRETCH
BACK EXTENSION
STRETCH PAGE 162

TAKE CARE
OTHER EXERCISES USING THE DEEP ABDOMINAL STABILISERS ARE BETTER OPTIONS IF YOU HAVE A BACK PROBLEM (SEE THE BACK IN ACTION PROGRAM ON PAGE 172).

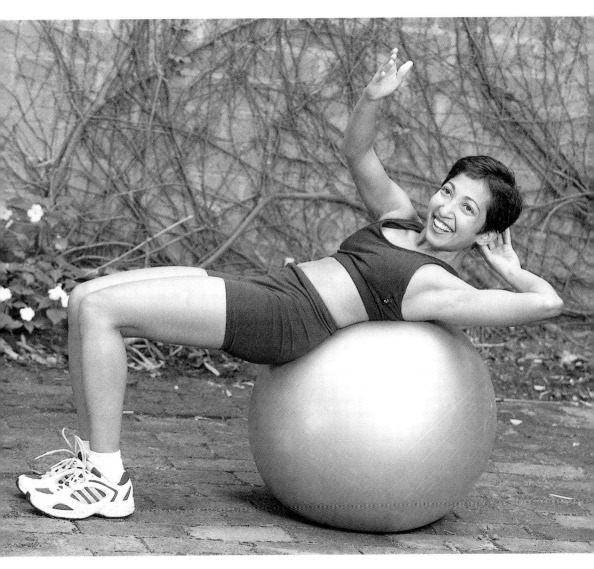

roll away

work your abs from the inside out

Starting position
- Kneel upright.
- Place your hands on the ball at arm's length in front of you.

Action
- Draw your shoulder blades back and down.
- Set your abdominals and tighen your gluteals, ie tuck in your butt.
- Roll the ball away, keeping your body in alignment as it inclines forward.
- Your forearms should be leaning on the ball.
- Keep your back straight and your butt tucked in.
- Hold for 10 slow counts, breathing normally.

Decrease the challenge
- Roll out and slowly back again without holding.

Increase the challenge
- Roll the ball a little further away.
- Hold the position while you roll the ball slightly, and slowly, from side to side.

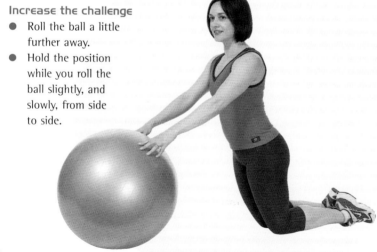

TRAINER TIPS

AIM FOR YOUR TORSO TO FORM A STRAIGHT LINE FROM YOUR KNEES TO SHOULDERS.

BE SURE TO ROLL OFF YOUR KNEES ONTO THE SOFT TISSUE OF YOUR THIGH, JUST ABOVE THE KNEES. THIS IS WHY YOUR FEET COME OFF THE FLOOR.

IF YOUR KNEES ARE UNCOMFORTABLE TRY KNEELING ON A THIN CUSHION OR ROLLED UP TOWEL.

STRETCH

KNEELING BACK STRETCH PAGE 145

TAKE CARE

AVOID HYPEREXTENSION AS IN THE SECOND PHOTOGRAPH OPPOSITE.

ARCHING YOUR BACK MEANS YOU ARE NOT WORKING YOUR ABS AND YOU ARE PLACING YOUR BACK AT RISK.

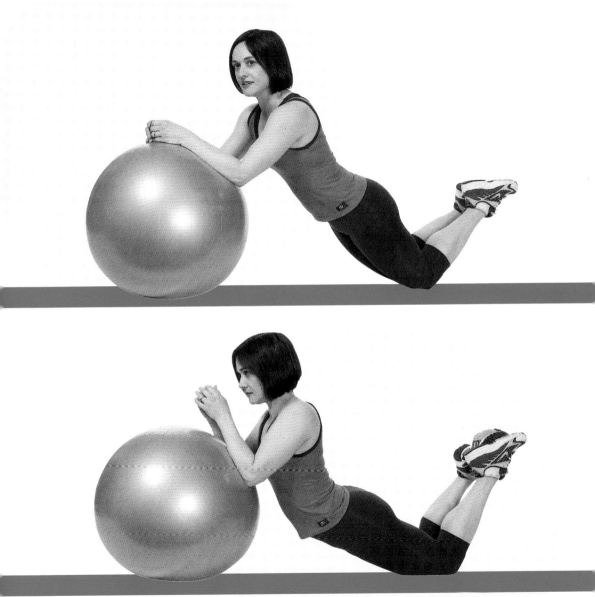

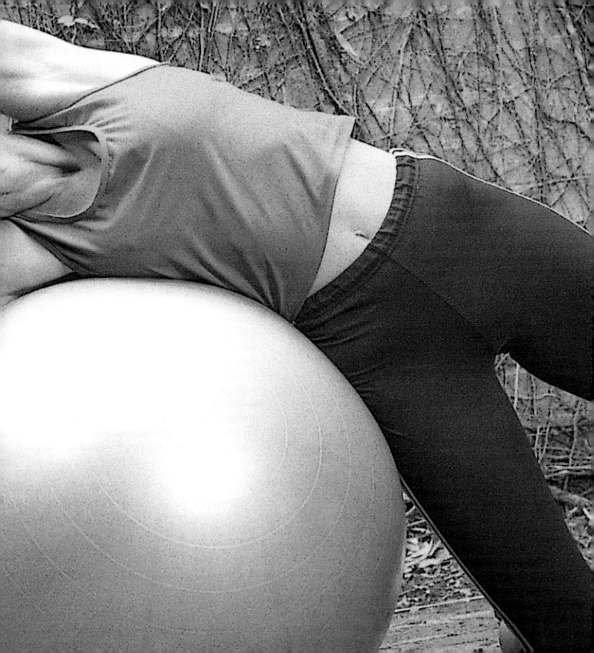

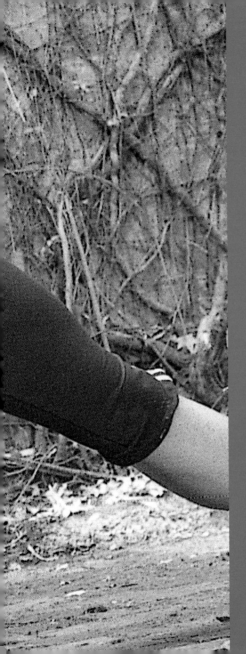

Attack your body from every angle.

Lying sideways over the exercise ball
provides a highly effective position to
strengthen the lateral muscles of the torso, hips
and thighs. The ball supports the body,
allowing for an intense focus on the waist,
butt and thighs. It also provides instability
in the side lean, which in turn fine-tunes
the stability of the back and pelvis.

Blitz the muscles on the side of your body
for well-proportioned, all-round perfection.

sideways on the ball

side leg raise

a get-tough workout for your thigh, buttocks and waist

Starting position
- Kneel on the floor and push your ball in under your left thigh.
- Lie over the ball and straighten out your right leg.
- Take a moment to move your left knee to a comfortable position.
- Lying over the ball, rest your head in your left hand.
- Keeping your knee straight, raise your leg off the ground to the horizontal position.

Action
Thigh raise and lower
- Keeping your leg extended, lower your right foot to the ground then raise your leg back to hip height.
- 15 reps x 3, each side

Decrease the challenge
- Lie on your side on the floor for an easier option.

Increase the challenge
- Increase number of reps or sets.
- Perform this exercise holding a weight in your top arm, resting it on your thigh as close to the knee as possible.
- Hold the straight leg at the top for five counts with every raise.

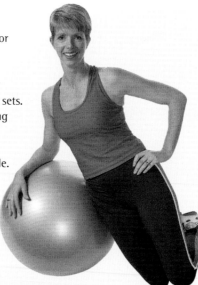

TRAINER TIPS
SET YOUR ABDOMINALS TO GIVE THE THIGH A STRONG AND STABLE WORKING BASE.

KEEP YOUR LEG LONG AND STRAIGHT. SLIGHTLY RELAXING THE KNEE WILL DECREASE THE INTENSITY OF THE BUTTOCK WORKOUT.

STRETCH
EXTENDED SIDE STRETCH PAGE 149

TAKE CARE
IF YOUR WEIGHT-BEARING KNEE IS UNCOMFORTABLE, PUT A CUSHION OR ROLLED-UP TOWEL UNDER IT FOR PADDING, OR LIE ON YOUR SIDE ON THE FLOOR.

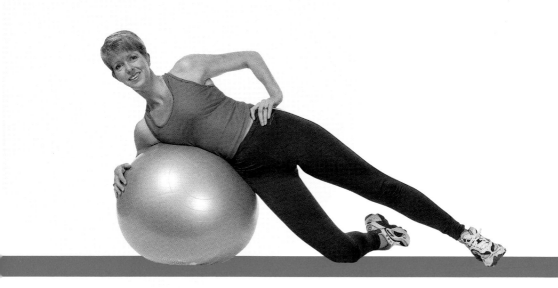

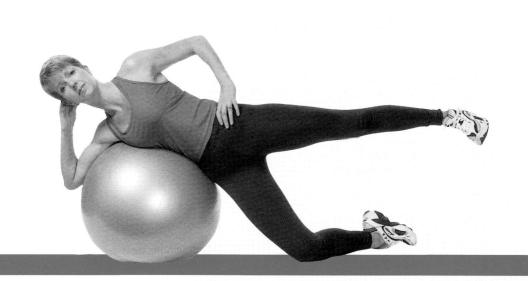

lateral curl

extra focus on obliques

This exercise is for people who are confident with ball training and are looking for more challenge. It can be a little awkward at first but persevere for an excellent complement to other abdominal training.

Starting position
- Kneel on your left knee with your right foot forward (the 'propose' position).
- Place the ball against your left thigh.
- Tuck your left toes under so you can 'walk' up the ball, bringing the left knee up off the floor.
- Walk your hips up as high as possible on the ball.
- Your foward knee should be bent with the foot flat on the floor in front.
- The left knee should be bent with the foot behind your body, leaning into the ball of the foot for balance.
- Rest your left hand beside you on the ball with your right hand behind your head.

Action
Side curl
- Set your abdominals.
- Roll your left side up off the ball.
- Roll back down over the ball.
- 10 reps x 2, each side

TRAINER TIPS
STRONGLY SET YOUR ABDOMINALS TO PROVIDE A STABLE BASE FOR THE LATERAL FLEXION OF YOUR TORSO.

ALTHOUGH THE LOWER ARM IS SUPPORTING YOU, RESIST THE TEMPTATION TO PUSH UP WITH IT.

STRETCH
KNEELING SIDE STRETCH PAGE 148

TAKE CARE
KEEP YOUR NECK ALIGNED WITH YOUR SPINE AND AVOID PULLING ON YOUR HEAD.

PERFORM THIS EXERCISE ON A NON-SLIP SURFACE.

Decrease the challenge

● Start in the same position but keep the lower knee on the floor. You will still be able
to curl sideways off the ball but with a more stable base, allowing you to focus on
your technique and form.

Increase the challenge

● Increase the number of reps or sets.
● Take the assisting arm off the ball and place it behind your head also.
● Walk your hip higher up the ball.

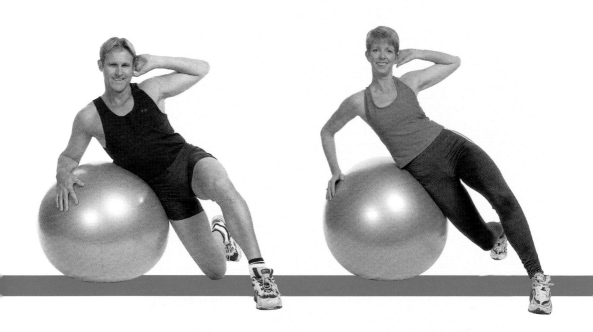

side lean

a leaning tower of strength

Starting position
- Kneel upright beside the ball. It should not be touching your thigh.
- Rest your forearm low on the ball close to your side.

Action
Lean sideways
- Set your abdominals.
- Draw your shoulder blades down and tighten your gluteals.
- Tilt your body sideways on a slight angle, leaning into the ball through the forearm.
- Keep your body in a straight line.
- The outer knee may come slightly off the floor.
- Hold for 10 counts.
- 3 reps, each side

Decrease the challenge
- Hold the position for 5 counts, then slowly build up as your endurance increases.

Increase the challenge
- Hold the position for longer.

TRAINER TIPS

KEEP YOUR SHOULDER BLADES DRAWN BACK AND DOWN.

DO NOT LET YOUR HIPS TILT TO EITHER SIDE AND BE SURE THEY DO NOT TOUCH THE BALL.

CHECK YOUR ALIGNMENT IN A MIRROR.

STRETCH

KNEELING SIDE STRETCH PAGE 148

TAKE CARE

THIS EXERCISE REQUIRES SOUND SHOULDER STABILISATION AS WELL AS PELVIC AND LUMBAR CONTROL. IT MAY BE INAPPROPRIATE IF YOU HAVE A KNEE, NECK OR SHOULDER PROBLEM.

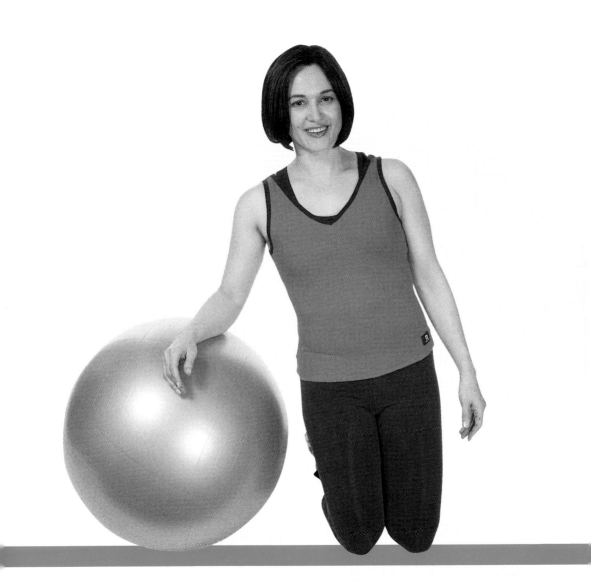

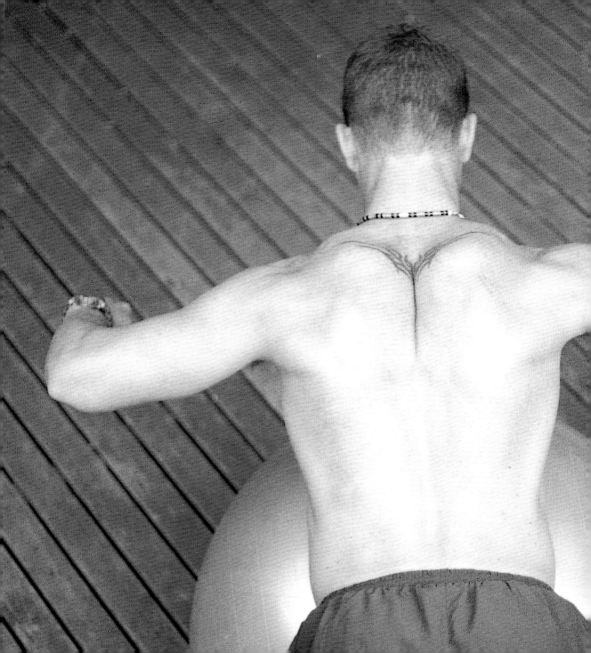

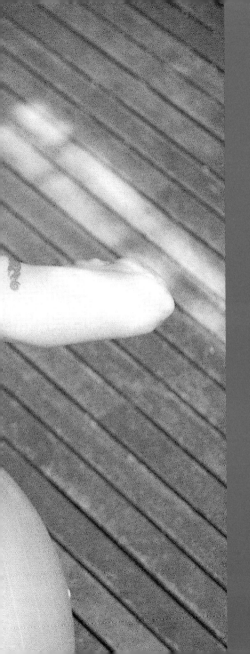

When you are in the prone position you lie face-down on the exercise ball. This is the ideal position for strengthening all the posterior muscle groups vital for balance, posture and a strong, stable spine. The ball is equally effective for training the muscles of the upper and lower back and offers greater advantages over traditional back-strengthening approaches because:

• it provides support for the lumbar spine and pelvis

• it raises the body off the ground, allowing for full range of arm and leg movements

• the unstable environment incorporates the training of balance and spinal stabilisation as well as strengthening the posterior muscles.

In the prone position the ball is placed under the hips and lower abdomen. Start by getting used to this position and then enjoy a new range of exercises that provide a total back conditioning program. Get on the ball for a great look from behind.

prone on the ball

prone on the ball

getting started

The basic position is the same for strengthening the upper and lower back.

Starting position

- Kneel behind the ball and then roll forward and over it.
- Lie facing the floor with the ball under your hips and lower abdomen.
- Rest your hands lightly on the floor in front of the ball.
- Raise your chest to create a straight incline from your feet to your shoulders. Use your back muscles to hold your chest off the ball. Do not lean on your hands.
- Have the balls of your feet firmly on the ground. Balancing on your toes is too unstable.
- Keep your feet close together.

TRAINER TIPS

KEEP YOUR NECK IN A NEUTRAL POSITION (IN LINE WITH YOUR SPINE) BY LOOKING DOWN AT THE FLOOR.

THE LESS YOU USE YOUR ARMS THE MORE YOU STRENGTHEN YOUR BACK. EVENTUALLY YOU WILL BE ABLE TO PERFORM THE LEG EXERCISES WITH ONE OR BOTH HANDS OFF THE FLOOR.

TAKE CARE

AVOID EATING BEFORE EXERCISING IN GENERAL, BUT ESPECIALLY BEFORE LYING PRONE ON THE BALL.

PRONE EXERCISES ARE HARD WORK FOR YOUR BACK. TAKE FREQUENT RESTS AS REQUIRED. OMIT ANY POSITIONS THAT CAUSE PAIN.

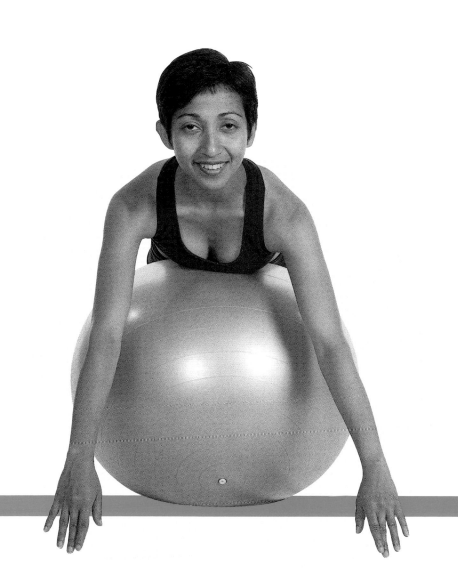

wide row

work your upper back

Starting position
- Use your level 1 weights.
- Prone on the ball.
- Hold your weights end to end on the floor in front of the ball.

Action
Raise and squeeze
- Squeezing your shoulder blades together, raise your arms out and up while bending your elbows to take the weights out in a wide arc.
- Lower the weights slowly down to the starting position in front of the ball.
- 15 reps x 3

Decrease the challenge
- Start by using one arm at a time.
- Progress to using both arms but no weights.

Increase the challenge
- Increase weights, number of reps or sets.
- Try the exercise with one leg straight and raised off the ground.

TRAINER TIPS
KEEP YOUR CHEST SLIGHTLY RAISED OFF THE BALL TO HELP STRENGTHEN THE BACK MUSCLES.

FOCUS ON DRAWING YOUR SHOULDER BLADES TOGETHER.

RELAX YOUR NECK AND TUCK YOUR CHIN IN. LOOKING UP ALL THE TIME MAY CAUSE NECK DISCOMFORT.

REMEMBER THE BALLS OF YOUR FEET SHOULD BE FIRMLY ON THE FLOOR AND CLOSE TOGETHER.

STRETCH
UPPER BACK
STRETCH PAGE 159

TAKE CARE
LISTEN TO YOUR BODY. IF THE EXERCISE CAUSES DISCOMFORT, REST FREQUENTLY BY GETTING OFF THE BALL AND ROLLING IT OUT IN FRONT TO STRETCH.

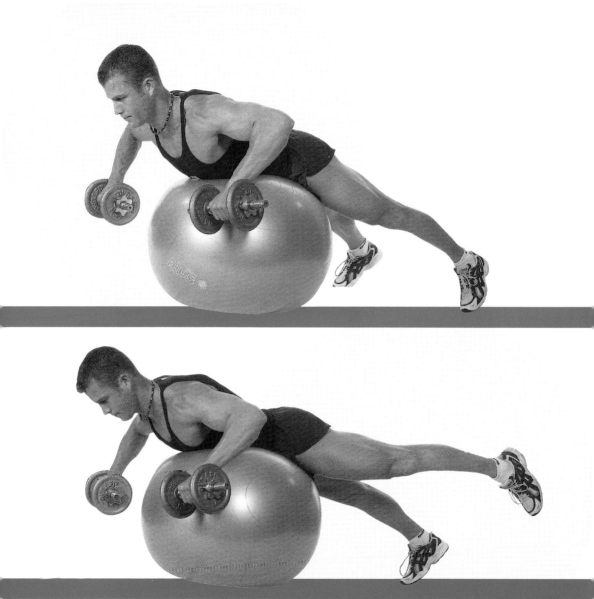

prone low row
postural perfection

Starting position
- Hold a level 1 weight in each hand.
- Prone over the ball.
- Upper arms high and tucked in close to your ribs.
- Bend your elbows with weights close to your hips.
- Draw your shoulder blades back.

Action
Reach and pull back
- Reach foward and down towards the floor, extending your elbows.
- Pull back up, bending your elbows and drawing your shoulder blades back again.
- 15 reps x 2

Decrease the challenge
- Use no weights to start with.
- Perform the exercise with one arm at a time.

Increase the challenge
- Increase weights, number of reps or sets.
- Repeat the exercise with alternating leg raises.

TRAINER TIPS
HOLD YOUR CHEST SLIGHTLY
UP AND OFF THE BALL AND
RESIST THE TEMPTATION TO
LOWER YOUR CHEST EACH
TIME THE WEIGHTS GO
TOWARDS THE FLOOR.

BE SURE TO USE THE
MUSCLES BEHIND YOUR
SHOULDERS AND IN YOUR
UPPER BACK TO DRAW YOUR
ARMS BACK AND UP.

KEEP YOUR ARMS TUCKED
IN CLOSE TO YOUR SIDE.

STRETCH
UPPER BACK
STRETCH PAGE 159

TAKE CARE
LOOK DOWN TO AVOID
STRAINING YOUR NECK.

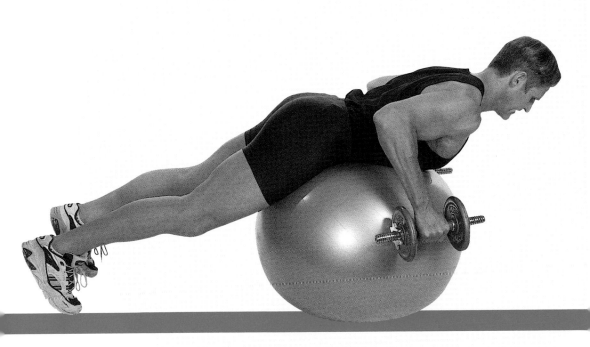

triceps press back

sculpt your back and arms

Starting position
- Use your level 1 weights.
- Prone over the ball, feet on the floor and chest slightly raised.
- Hold your weights by your hips with your elbows high and close to your sides.

Action
Press with the triceps
- Straighten your elbows to press the weights towards the ceiling.
- Bend your elbows to lower your hands back to the ball.
- 15 reps x 3

Decrease the challenge
- Use no weight to start with.

Increase the challenge
- Increase weights, number of reps or sets.
- Combine the prone low row and triceps press back in one movement. Start with your elbows high and flexed. Reach to the floor. Pull slowly back and up. Press the weights upwards to straighten your elbows. Lower the weights back to the bent elbow position, ready to start again.

TRAINER TIPS
RELAX YOUR NECK.

KEEP YOUR ELBOWS
HIGH AND TUCKED IN.

SLOW CONTROLLED
MOVEMENT IS IMPORTANT.
AVOID SWINGING AND JOLTING
TO PREVENT STRAINING.

STRETCH
TRICEPS STRETCH PAGE 160

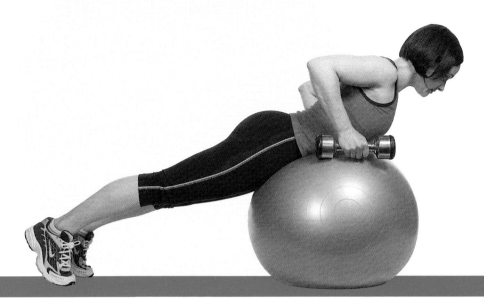

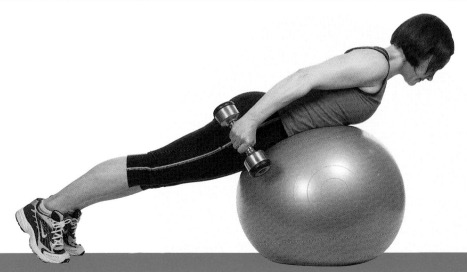

prone push back

honing in on your upper back

Starting position
- Hold your level 1 weight close to the floor in front of the ball.
- Prone over the ball, feet on the floor and chest slightly raised.
- Extend arms towards the floor in front of the ball.

Action
Push up and back
- Raise arms back and upwards, taking your hands to hip height.
- Slightly turn your palms inwards to gently squeeze your shoulder blades together.
- Lower your arms back to the starting position.
- 15 reps x 2

Decrease the challenge
- Use no weights to start with.
- Perform the exercise one arm at a time.

Increase the challenge
- Increase weights, number of reps or sets.
- Bring your feet together.
- Hold one leg off the floor for the first set. Change legs for the second.

TRAINER TIPS

KEEP YOUR CHEST SLIGHTLY UP OFF THE BALL, BUT RELAX YOUR NECK.

FOCUS ON CONTRACTING THE MUSCLES BETWEEN YOUR SHOULDERS.

AS YOU TURN YOUR HANDS INWARDS AT THE TOP, PULL YOUR SHOULDER BLADES TOWARDS EACH OTHER.

STRETCH
UPPER BACK
STRETCH PAGE 159

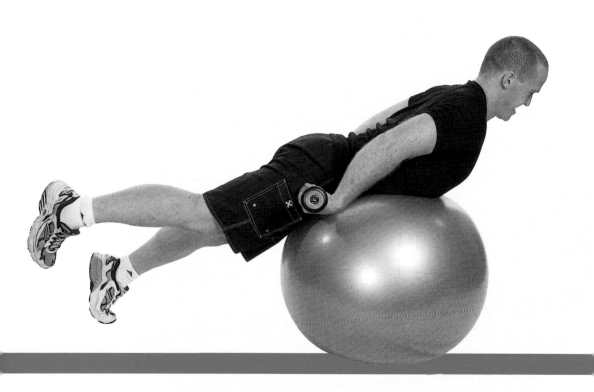

107

back extension

back in action

Starting position
- Prone over the ball, feet on the floor and chest lowered.
- Rest your hands lightly on the ball.

Action
Extend back and up
- Slowly raise your chest up off the ball.
- Raise your arms off the ball sideways, keeping your elbows slightly bent.
- Lower your arms and chest slowly.
- 10 reps x 2

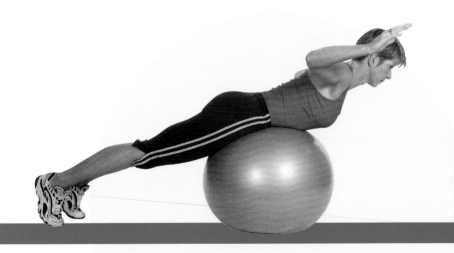

TRAINER TIPS

SQUEEZE YOUR SHOULDER BLADES TOGETHER AS YOU RAISE YOUR BACK AND ARMS.

FOCUS ON USING YOUR BACK MUSCLES TO RAISE YOUR CHEST.

YOU DO NOT NEED TO RAISE TOO HIGH. A SMALL AMOUNT OF EXTENSION OFF THE BALL IS BENEFICIAL.

KEEP THE MOVEMENT SLOW AND CONTROLLED.

STRETCH
KNEELING BACK STRETCH PAGE 145

TAKE CARE
EXTENSION OVER THE BALL CAN BE TOUGH. WORK ONLY WITHIN YOUR RANGE OF COMFORT AND BE PATIENT. SLOW PROGRESSION IS WISE.

Decrease the challenge
- Keep your hands lightly on the ball as you raise your chest.

Increase the challenge
- Raise your chest up off the ball holding your arms out to the side, elbows bent.
- Reach your arms forward.
- Pull your arms back, drawing your shoulder blades together.
- Lower your chest back onto the ball.

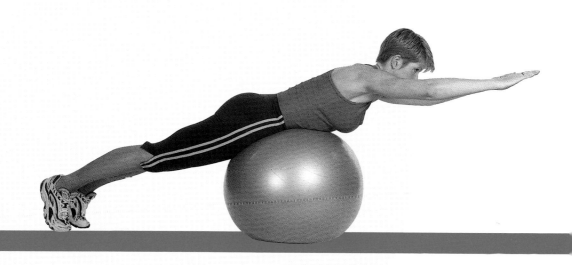

prone leg raise

lower back and butt

Starting position
- Prone over the ball, fingertips and feet on the floor and chest slightly raised.

Action
- Raise one leg up to hip height and hold for two counts.
- Lower slowly.
- 15 reps x 2 each side

Decrease the challenge
- Do fewer reps on each leg.
- Don't hold at the top, keep your leg moving.
- Alternate legs instead of 15 reps on one side then the other.

Increase the challenge
- Increase number of reps or sets.
- Take your hands off the floor and rest them lightly on the ball or by your hips.
- Raise and hold for five counts before lowering down.

TRAINER TIPS

KEEP THE WEIGHT OFF YOUR HANDS.

KEEP YOUR KNEE COMPLETELY STRAIGHT.

FOCUS ON CONTRACTING YOUR GLUTEALS TO RAISE THE LEG.

STRETCH

GLUTEAL STRETCH PAGE 141

TAKE CARE

KEEP YOUR NECK ALIGNED WITH YOUR SPINE TO AVOID NECK STRAIN.

IF YOU FEEL DISCOMFORT DISCONTINUE THE EXERCISE.

IF YOUR BACK IS WEAK, TAKE FREQUENT RESTS OFF THE BALL, ROLLING IT FORWARD TO STRETCH YOUR BACK.

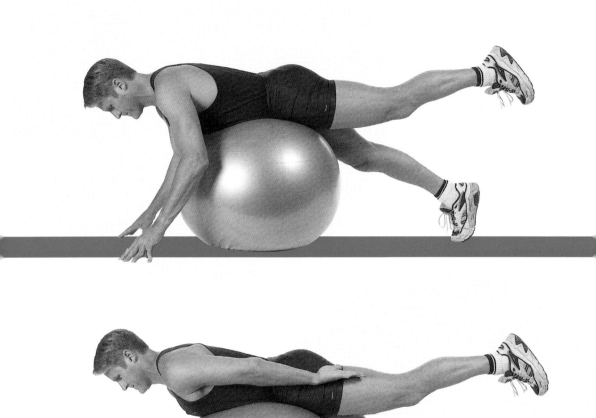

prone swim kick

balance and strength come together

Starting position

- Prone over the ball.
- Place your fingertips lightly on the floor for balance.
- Legs are raised and horizontal with straight knees.
- Your body should form a straight line from shoulders to toes.

Action

Kick

- Kick your legs, keeping your body horizontal.
- Do small strong kicks for two minutes.
- Follow with larger kicks for one minute so feet alternately touch the floor.

TRAINER TIPS

BEFORE STARTING TO KICK FIND THE BALANCE POINT WHERE YOU COULD ALMOST BALANCE WITH YOUR HANDS OFF THE FLOOR. THIS IS THE IDEAL STARTING POSITION.

KEEP YOUR KNEES STRAIGHT.

KICK FROM YOUR GLUTEALS.

KEEP YOUR NECK IN LINE WITH YOUR SPINE BY LOOKING AT THE FLOOR MOST OF THE TIME.

STRETCH

DRAPE PAGE 150

Decrease the challenge

● Do small straight leg kicks for one minute.

Increase the challenge

● Kick with one hand off the floor. Alternate hands each 10 kicks. This will further challenge your stability and balance.

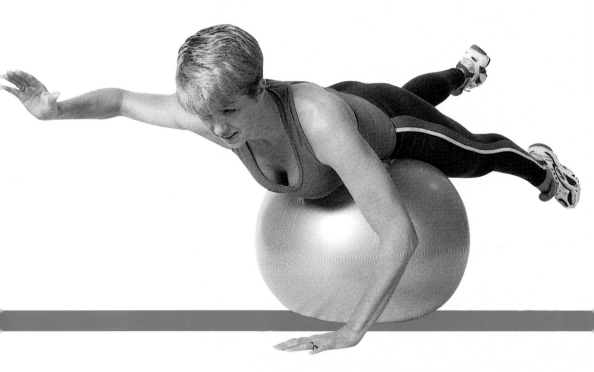

pike
straight and strong

Starting position
- Prone over the ball with legs extended so your body is horizontal from shoulders to toes.
- Keep your legs very straight and your heels together.
- Place your fingertips lightly on the floor for balance.

Action
Lower and raise
- Simultaneously lower your legs and chest slowly towards the floor.
- Raise legs and chest slowly back to the horizontal position.
- 15 reps x 2

Decrease the challenge
- Lower and raise your legs 5 times slowly.
- Then lower and raise your chest 5 times slowly.

Increase the challenge
- Lower then raise chest and legs and hold this position while slowly opening and closing the legs in a scissor motion.

TRAINER TIPS

DO NOT USE YOUR ARMS.

KEEP YOUR KNEES STRAIGHT AND LEGS LONG.

CONTRACT YOUR GLUTEALS AS YOU RAISE YOUR LEGS.

KEEP THE ACTION SLOW AND STRONG IN BOTH DIRECTIONS.

STRETCH

SPINAL ROTATION PAGE 142

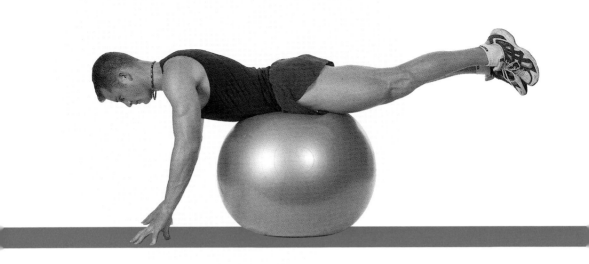

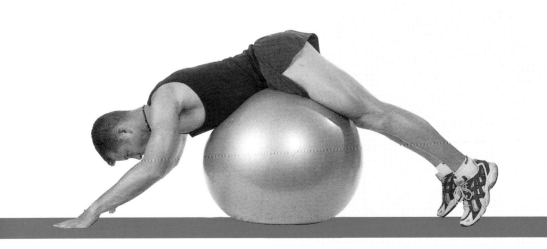

raise and reach

back, butt and balance

Starting position
- Prone over the ball.
- Arms straight and in front of the ball.

Action
Arm and leg raise
- Raise one hand out in front of you to shoulder height.
- Simultaneously, raise the opposite leg up to hip height.
- Hold for 5 counts.
- Lower your hand and foot to the floor.
- Repeat on the other side.
- 15 reps each side

Decrease the challenge
- Do 10 reps each side.
- Raise alternating arms alone, then alternating legs alone.

Increase the challenge
- Use your level 1 weights.
- Make this a three-limb raise. Take the second arm back towards your hip as you raise the opposite arm and leg. This creates an alternating paddling action with the arms.

Go harder
- Reach both arms up and forward as you raise alternating legs.

TRAINER TIPS
TUCK YOUR CHIN IN TO AVOID STRAINING YOUR NECK.

KEEP YOUR ELBOWS AND KNEES STRAIGHT.

KEEP YOUR CHEST UP AND YOUR OTHER HAND OFF THE FLOOR TO FURTHER STRENGTHEN YOUR BACK.

STRETCH
KNEELING BACK STRETCH PAGE 145

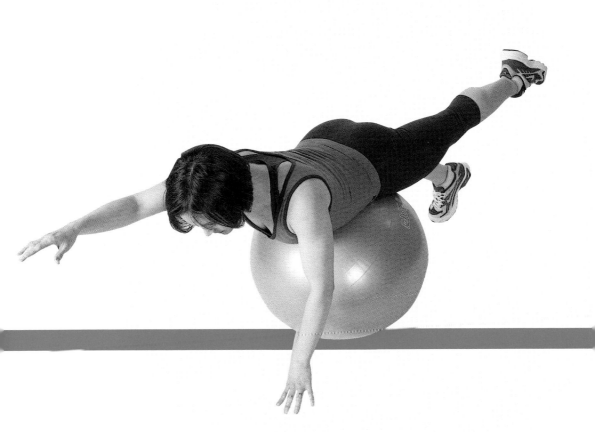

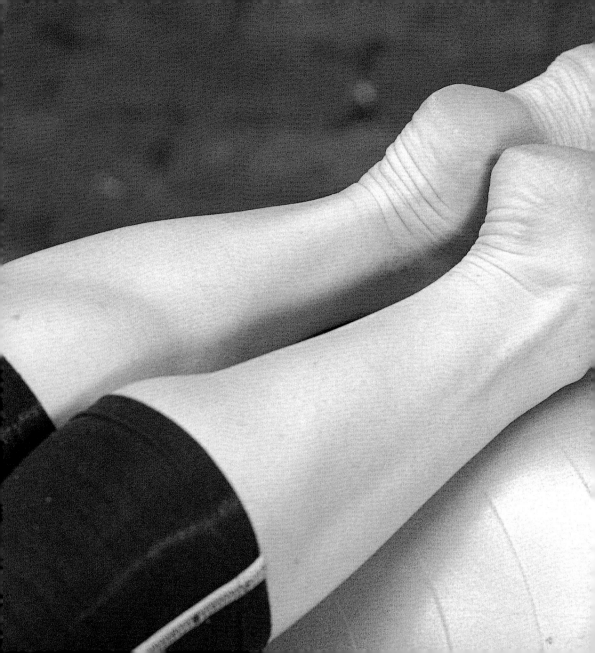

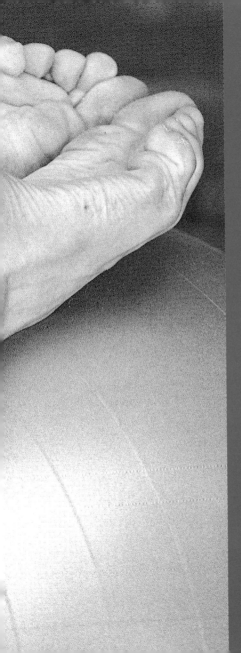

The forward prone position provides a fabulous workout that not only firms your torso but also strengthens the deep stabilising muscles around your shoulders, pelvis and spine.

When you walk out on your hands into forward prone, the ball no longer supports the lower back and pelvis, so the abdominal stabilisers become vital players. This position also requires significant shoulder strength.

It is easy to alter the intensity of these exercises by simply walking your hands further out from, or keeping them closer to, the ball. The ball may be positioned anywhere between under your thighs to under your toes. The closer it is to your feet, the more effort is required to prevent your lower back from swaying. These longer levered exercises require more strength and control in both the upper body and the deep stabilisers of the spine.

Make sure you work at a distance from the ball where you can maintain good movement control and spinal position. If your lower back is swaying or your upper back is rounding, step your hands back to shorten the lever. Drawing your lower abdomen towards your spine to set the deep supporting muscles is a high priority in all forward prone exercises. Remember, quality not quantity.

Train in this challenging position for a stellar workout and a powerful, defined physique.

forward prone on the ball

push-up
a fresh challenge to an old favourite

Starting position
- Kneel on the floor, then roll forward over the ball to the horizontal prone position.
- Walk forward slowly on your hands. The distance you walk out from the ball determines the intensity of the exercise. Start with the ball under your thighs or knees.
- Set your abdominals to keep your back straight and well supported. Don't let your back sway.
- Keep your knees straight.

Action
Push up
- Bend your elbows, slowly lowering your chest towards the floor.
- Push slowly back up.
- 10 reps x 3

Decrease the challenge
- Start out with the ball under your hips. Gradually walk your hands forward as you get stronger, always emphasising good technique.
- The wall push-up (page 62) is an excellent modification for this exercise.

Increase the challenge
- Walk your hands further away from the ball to increase the intensity.

Go harder
- Place just your toes on the ball to be at your longest lever option.
- Different arm positions alter the muscle focus. Bringing your hands closer together emphasises the triceps and further challenges stability.

TRAINER TIPS
AVOID LOCKING YOUR ELBOWS AT THE TOP OF THE MOVEMENT BY STOPPING JUST BEFORE THEY ARE FULLY EXTENDED.

IF YOU ARE UNABLE TO MAINTAIN A STRAIGHT BACK AND GOOD TECHNIQUE, WALK YOUR HANDS BACK A STEP AND PROGRESS FORWARD AGAIN AS YOU GET STRONGER.

STRETCH
PECS STRETCH PAGE 147

TAKE CARE
THIS EXERCISE IS INAPPROPRIATE IF YOU HAVE A SHOULDER, NECK OR BACK PROBLEM.

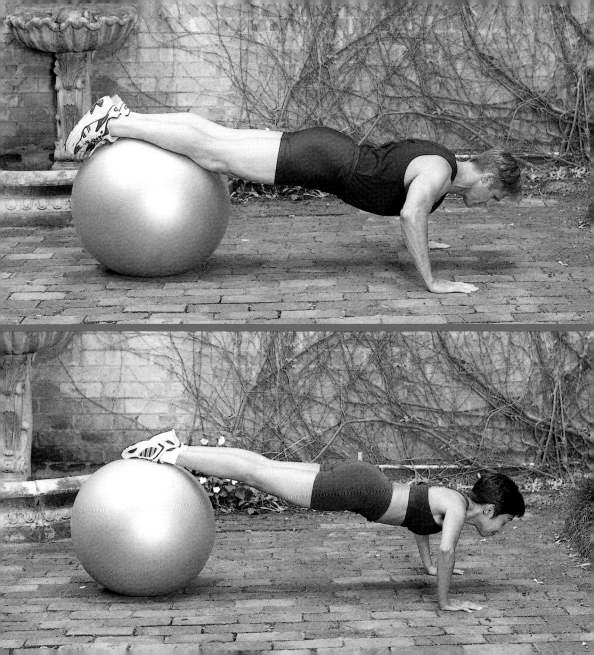

plank
long and lean

An endurance test. Increase the holding time of this one as you get stronger.

Starting position
- Kneel on your hands and knees.
- Rest your shins and the front of your feet on the ball behind you.

Action
Roll out and hold
- Set your abdominals.
- Slowly roll the ball back to raise your feet and straighten your knees.
- Maintain this horizontal position for 10 counts.
- Roll back to return to the kneeling position.
- Repeat x 4

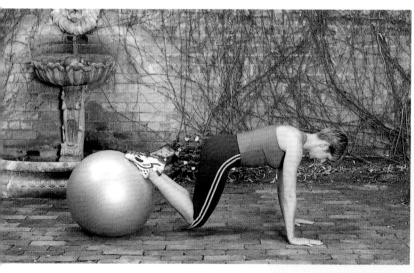

TRAINER TIPS

SET YOUR ABDOMINALS TO KEEP YOUR BACK STRAIGHT.

ROLL OUT AND BACK SLOWLY.

KEEP YOUR KNEES AND BACK STRAIGHT WHILE YOU ARE HORIZONTAL.

BREATHE NORMALLY WHILE YOU HOLD THE POSITION.

AVOID ROUNDING YOUR UPPER BACK.

STRETCH
ROCK AND ROLL PAGE 144

Decrease the challenge

● Slowly roll out to the horizontal position and then back in without holding.
● Gradually increase the hold time.

Increase the challenge

● Keeping your pelvis square to the floor, try rolling the ball slightly side to side while in the horizontal position.

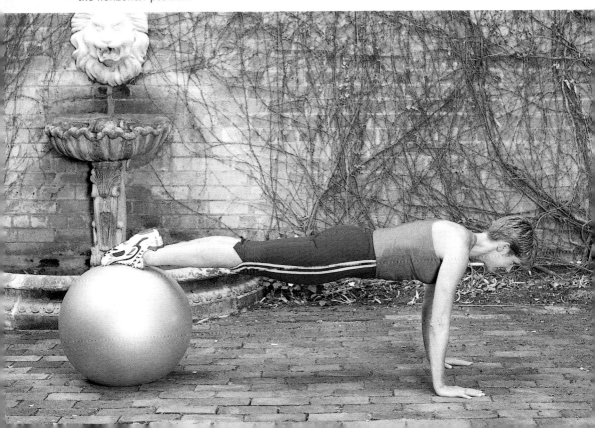

prone tuck

a mean abdominal workout

A toughie, combining inner and outer strength for smooth controlled movement.

Starting position
● Hands on the floor, feet on the ball (the horizontal plank position).

Action
Tuck in and out
● Set your abdominals to keep your back flat.
● Roll the ball in to bring your knees in under your hips.
● Slowly roll back to the horizontal plank position.
● Do not let your back sway or your bottom stick up.
● 5 slow reps.

Decrease the challenge
● Do the plank exercise (page 122) to start with.

Increase the challenge
● Increase the number of reps.
● Try a side tuck. Roll the ball slightly out to one side, bringing your knees around towards that side.

TRAINER TIPS

KEEP YOUR BACK FLAT AND YOUR HIPS LEVEL WITH YOUR SHOULDERS.

THIS EXERCISE IS BEST PERFORMED AS A CONTINUAL MOVEMENT ROLLING IN AND OUT, THE SLOWER THE BETTER.

STRETCH

ROCK AND ROLL PAGE 144

TAKE CARE

THE PRONE TUCK REQUIRES HIGH LEVELS OF STRENGTH AND CONTROL. IT IS INAPPROPRIATE FOR ANY ONE WITH EXISTING INJURIES, OR THOSE NEW TO EXERCISE BALL TRAINING.

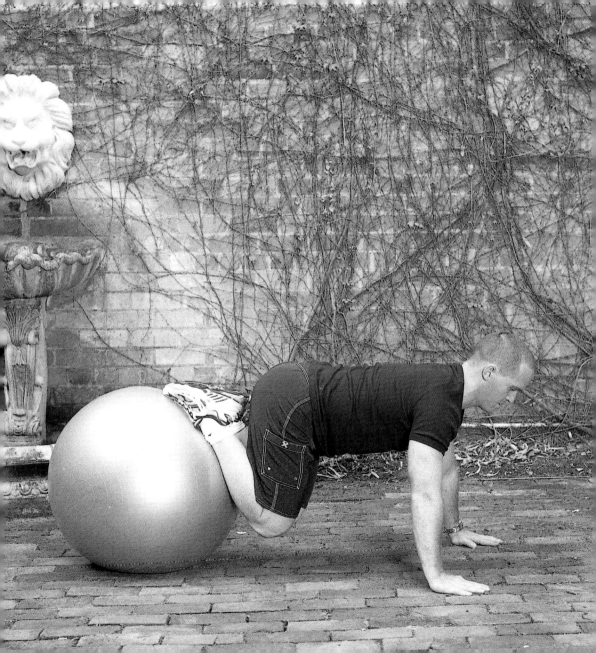

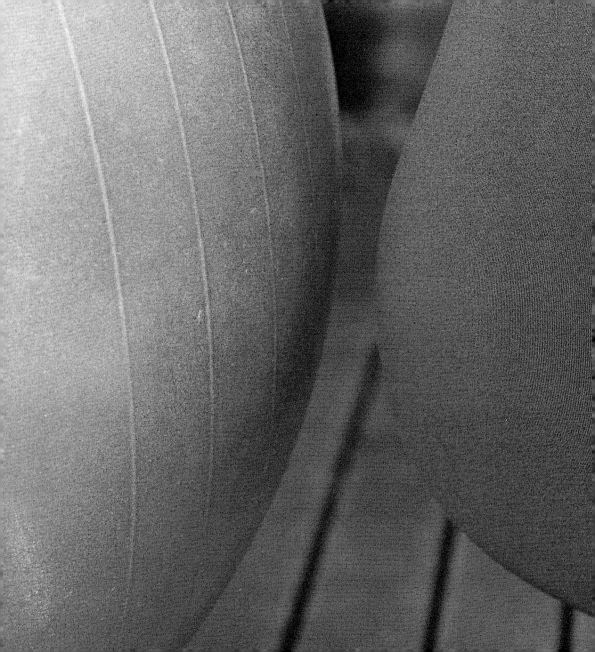

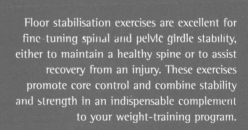

Floor stabilisation exercises are excellent for fine-tuning spinal and pelvic girdle stability, either to maintain a healthy spine or to assist recovery from an injury. These exercises promote core control and combine stability and strength in an indispensable complement to your weight-training program.

When you begin to do these exercises, rest your arms on the floor. Next try taking your forearms off the ground. Later you can feel proud of your core stability when you are strong enough to perform them with both arms off the floor.

supine on the floor

one leg lower

an excellent stabiliser

Starting position
- Supine on the floor, arms beside you.
- Rest your legs on top of the ball, with hips and knees bent to 90 degrees.
- Make sure the ball is right up against the back of your thighs.
- Focus on the neutral position of your lower back and keep your pelvis flat and square to the floor.

Action
- Set your abdominals.
- Slowly lower one leg to the floor and return it to the ball.
- Keep your back and pelvis in the neutral position.
- Repeat with the other leg.
- 10 reps each side

Decrease the challenge
- Bend your knee so your toes touch the floor just beside the ball. This shortens the lever and places less load on the spine and pelvis.

Increase the challenge
- Perform this exercise with your arms crossed over your chest.

TRAINER TIPS

DO NOT LET YOUR BACK ARCH UP OFF THE FLOOR OR YOUR PELVIS ROTATE.

KEEP THE OTHER LEG COMPLETELY RELAXED ON THE BALL.

KEEP YOUR HEAD ON THE FLOOR.

STRETCH

ROLL AND REACH PAGE 138

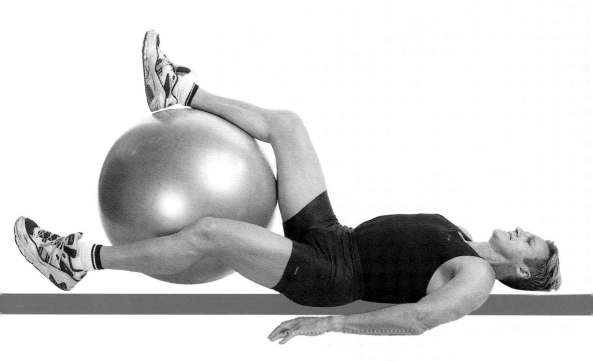

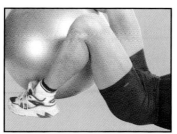

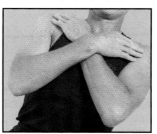

the clock

finely tuned core control

This exercise provides a subtle but very effective way to fine-tune deep abdominal awareness.

Starting position
- Supine on the floor.
- Relax your legs on top of the ball.
- Bend your hips and knees to 90 degrees.
- Make sure the ball is right up against your thighs.

Action
- Imagine your feet are the hands of a clock and the starting position is at the 12 o'clock position.
- Slowly roll to the right to the 10 past 2 position.
- Using your deep abdominals, particularly on the opposite side, roll the ball back to the 12 o'clock position.
- Repeat slowly x 10
- Slowly roll to the left to the 10 to 10 position and back to 12 o'clock.
- Repeat slowly x 10

Decrease the challenge
- Roll only to 5 past 1 and 5 to 11 to start with.
- Aim for quality, not quantity.

Increase the challenge
- Take your forearms off the floor.
- Try reaching your arms to the ceiling or crossing them over your chest.

TRAINER TIPS

ROLL TO THE POINT WHERE YOU STILL HAVE CONTROL AND THE OPPOSITE HIP IS ON THE FLOOR BUT FEELS LIKE IT IS ABOUT TO LIFT OFF.

FOCUS ON CONTRACTING YOUR DEEP ABDOMINALS TO DRIVE THE MOVEMENT BACK TO THE 12 O'CLOCK POSITION.

PERFORM SLOWLY FOR OPTIMAL BENEFITS.

THIS EXERCISE MAY BE FRUSTRATING AT FIRST UNTIL YOU ARE MORE AWARE OF YOUR DEEPER MUSCLES. BE PATIENT, IT WILL BE WORTH IT.

STRETCH
SUPINE ROCK PAGE 138

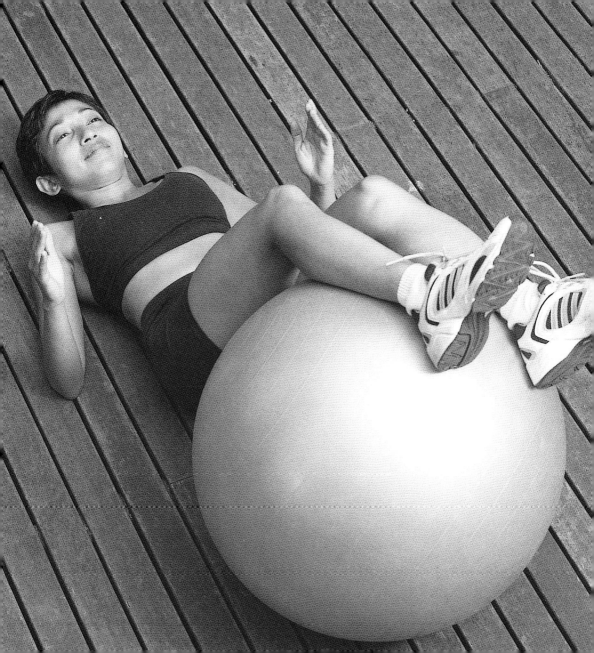

hamstring lift and roll

test how stable you really are

Starting position
- Supine on the floor.
- Arms resting by your side.
- Heels on top of the ball with your toes pulled back towards you.

Action
Lift and roll
- Raise your bottom off the floor.
- Roll the ball slowly in until your knees are above your hips.
- Roll back away.
- Lower your bottom back to the floor.
- 10 reps x 3

Decrease the challenge
- Raise your bottom very slightly off the floor.
- 5 reps x 3

Increase the challenge
- Take your arms off the floor and clasp your hands above your chest.
- Perform the exercise one leg at a time.

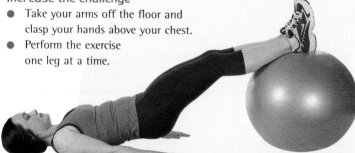

TRAINER TIPS
KEEP THE BACK OF YOUR HEELS RIGHT ON TOP OF THE BALL.

KEEP YOUR FEET PULLED BACK SO THAT THE SOLES OF YOUR SHOES DO NOT TOUCH THE BALL.

THE MORE YOU PUSH YOUR HEELS DOWN INTO THE BALL AS YOU ROLL IN AND OUT, THE MORE YOU WILL WORK YOUR HAMSTRINGS.

STRETCH
HAMSTRING STRETCH PAGE 140

132

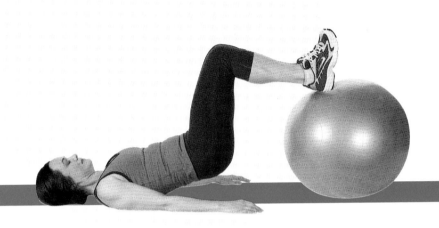

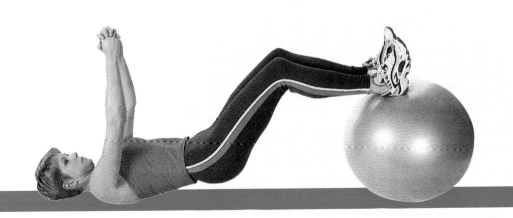

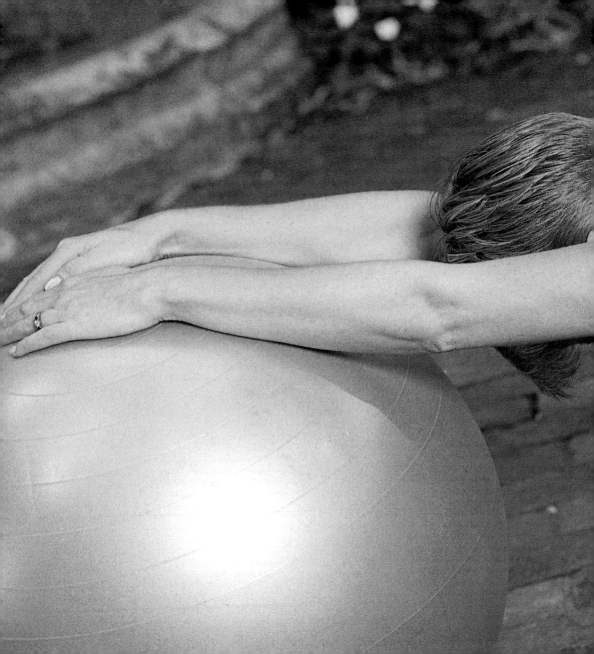

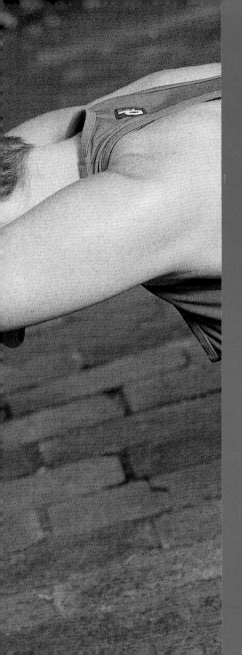

Mobility and flexibility are vital for a healthy body and mind.

Tight muscles cause discomfort, muscle imbalance, poor posture and injury. Gentle stretching keeps your muscles long and supple and releases tension in both body and mind.

The shape of the exercise ball allows for smooth flow of movement and comfortable positioning for a relaxing and reinvigorating cool-down. Perform these mobility and flexibility exercises for an effective finale to your training. You can also use them in their own right to provide a gentle workout that keeps you supple and calms your mind.

If you are in the habit of skimping on your stretching, you are not doing your body any favours. For a thorough workout and sensational results, give these important moves the time and attention they deserve. Your body will thank you.

mobility and flexibility

why stretch?

for health of body and mind

Mobility and flexibility exercises complement strength training and are an essential component of any workout. They decrease post-exercise soreness, assist injury prevention, improve posture and promote better quality of movement.

Gentle, rhythmical movements are used to keep your joints mobile and your body relaxed. Sustained stretches help maintain muscles that are long and flexible. Together they work to give you a supple, agile body and a calm, tranquil mind.

You may prefer to stretch each muscle group immediately after working it. For this purpose an appropriate stretch is indicated with each conditioning exercise. Or you can follow the relax and release programs on pages 182 and 183 or combine various stretches to create your own cool-down.

- take all the stretches to the point of slight tightness
- hold at that point for 40 to 60 seconds
- gently move further into the stretch if you feel the muscle release
- always perform cool-downs and stretching with a slow, calm approach
- always stretch without force
- if you feel any discomfort or you start shaking, you may be doing more harm than good

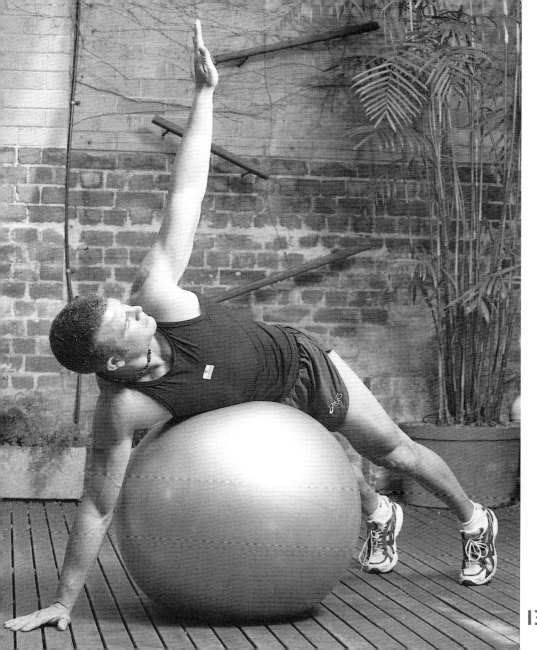

supine rock

- Lie supine on the floor with your feet resting on the ball.
- Gently rock the ball from side to side. Keep the rock slow and small to allow your back to relax and release.
- Continue for 40 to 60 seconds.

roll and reach

- Lie supine on the floor with your feet resting on the ball.
- Roll the ball in, bringing your knees towards your chest.
- Holding your knees, gently draw them closer to your chest.
- To take the stretch a little further, bring your chest up towards your knees.
- As you roll the ball away, reach your arms over your head to touch the floor and stretch your body from your fingers to your toes.
- Repeat 3 times slowly.

adductor stretch

- Lie supine on the floor with your feet resting on the ball and your soles turned towards each other.
- Allow your knees to fall apart.
- Roll the ball towards you, holding at the point where you feel a slight stretch in the inner thigh muscles.
- Hold for 40 to 60 seconds.

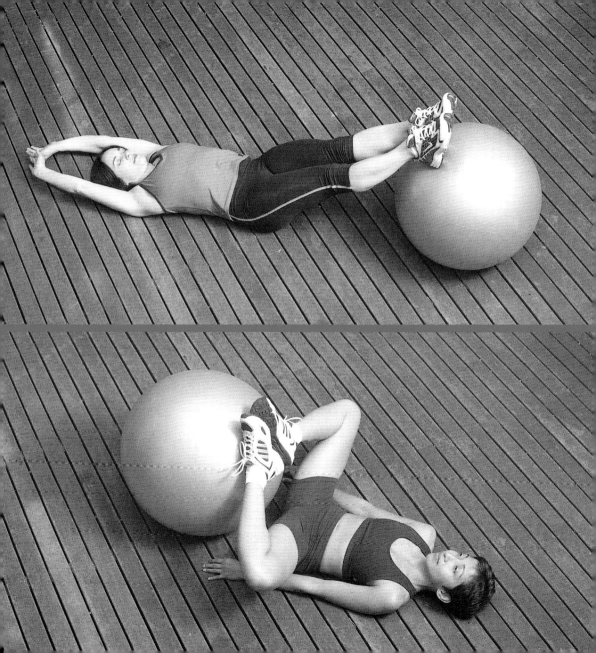

hamstring stretch

The hamstring stretch leads smoothly into the gluteal stretch. Do the hamstring stretch followed by the gluteal stretch on one side. Then perform both stretches on the other.

- Lie supine on the floor with your feet resting on the ball.
- Roll the ball in, bending your knees until they are directly above your hips.
- Hold one leg behind the thigh.
- Extend your leg towards the ceiling.
- Hold for 40 to 60 seconds.
- Keep your lower back and pelvis on the floor.
- You don't need to straighten your knee. Hold at the point where you feel a slight stretch.
- Holding the leg behind the thigh in the hamstring stretch puts less stress on the knee than holding the ankle.

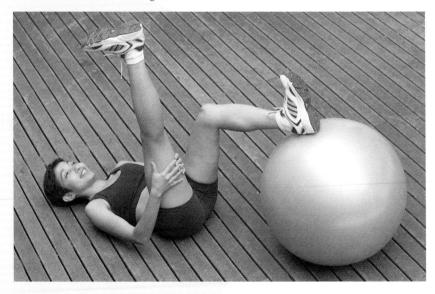

gluteal stretch

- Continue to hold the hamstring stretch position while you roll the ball away with your other leg.
- Cross your ankle over your thigh and let your knee fall outwards.
- Roll the ball towards you until you feel a stretch behind your hip in your buttock.
- Hold for 40 to 60 seconds.
- Tension in the gluteals can lead to back problems, so don't neglect this important stretch.

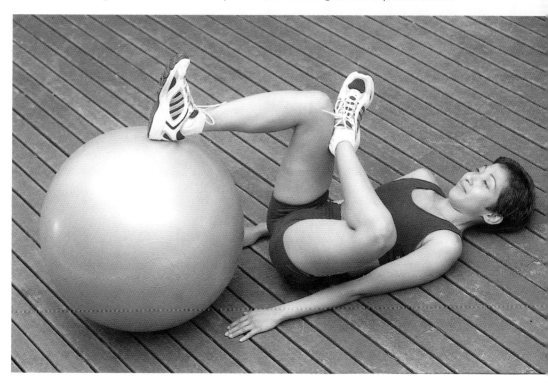

spinal rotation

- Lie supine with your knees bent and your feet flat on the floor.
- Hold the ball on the floor overhead.
- Roll your knees to the left side and the ball to the right.
- Take a slow deep breath and relax your back into the stretch as you exhale.
- Hold the stretch while you breathe normally for 40 to 60 seconds.
- Keep your feet on the floor as you slowly roll to the other side.
- Repeat twice to each side.

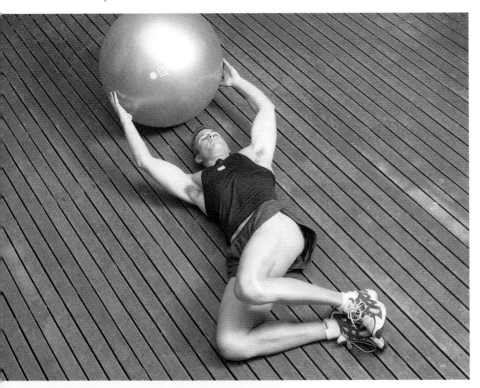

reach and release

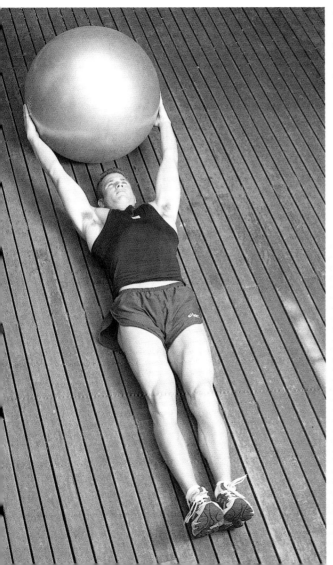

- Lie supine on the floor with your legs straight.
- Hold the ball on the floor overhead.
- Taking a deep breath, reach with your arms and roll the ball to stretch your body from your fingers to your toes.
- Relax as you exhale.
- Repeat 3 times.

rock and roll

This wonderful movement eases away tension and tightness in your back.

- Kneel on the floor and relax your forearms across the front of the ball. Rest your head on your hands.
- Roll your arms and the ball slowly from side to side, gently rotating through your middle back.
- Check that your back is flat and relaxed. If your upper back is rounded, move the ball further away to allow your back to relax down.
- Rock from side to side slowly.

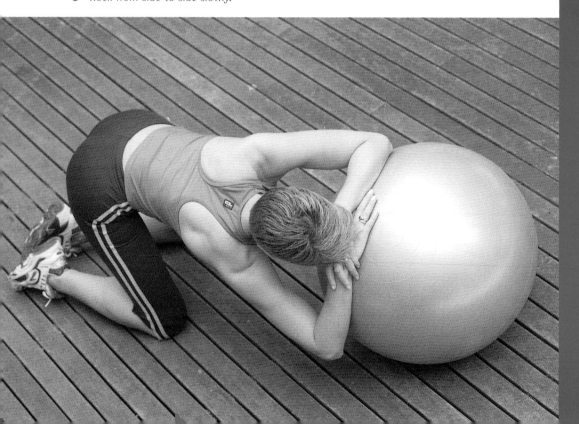

kneeling back stretch

- Keeping your back straight, sit back towards your heels as you roll the ball fowards.
- Elongate your torso from your fingers to your hips. You should feel a good stretch through your arms, back and buttocks.
- Roll up slowly into an upright kneeling position, starting at your lower back and finishing at your neck. Imagine you are rolling up one vertebra at a time.
- Repeat 3 times.

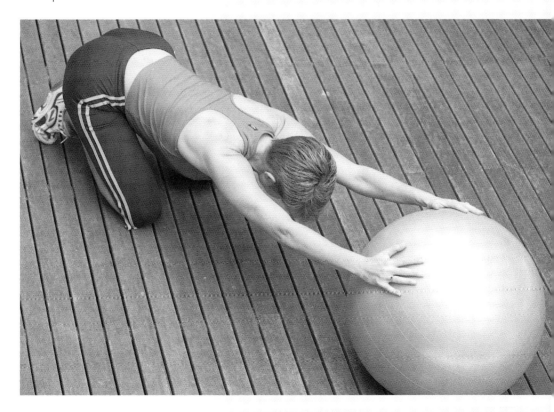

lats stretch

- Kneel behind the ball and place your right hand on the side of the ball.
- Roll the ball across your body to the left as you sit back towards your right heel.
- Push the ball slightly further across and away from you to feel a long stretch down your right side from your shoulder blade to your hip.
- Hold for 40 to 60 seconds.
- Repeat on the other side.

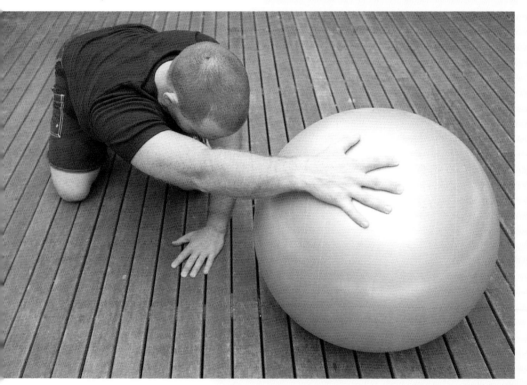

pecs stretch

- Kneel with the ball on your left side and your left hand resting on it.
- Lower your chest towards the floor, supporting your weight with your right hand.
- Turn away from the ball to feel a gentle stretch in the front of your shoulder and chest.
- Hold for 40 to 60 seconds.
- Repeat on the right side.

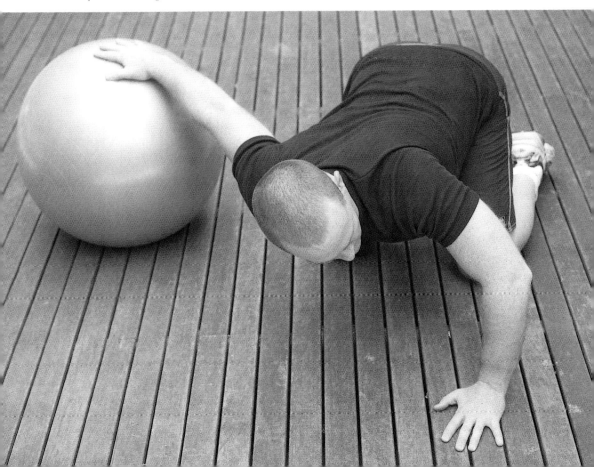

kneeling side stretch

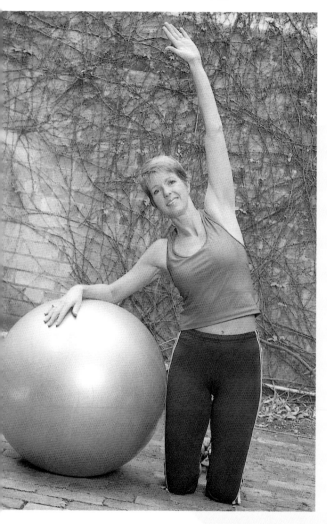

- Kneel with the ball against your left hip and thigh and rest your left forearm on top.
- Lean slightly over as you reach your right arm upwards.
- Hold for 40 to 60 seconds.
- Repeat on the other side.

extended side stretch

- Kneel with the ball against your left hip.
- Lie over the ball, extending your outer leg and reaching your right arm up and over to stretch sideways over the ball.
- Hold for 40 to 60 seconds.
- Repeat on the other side.

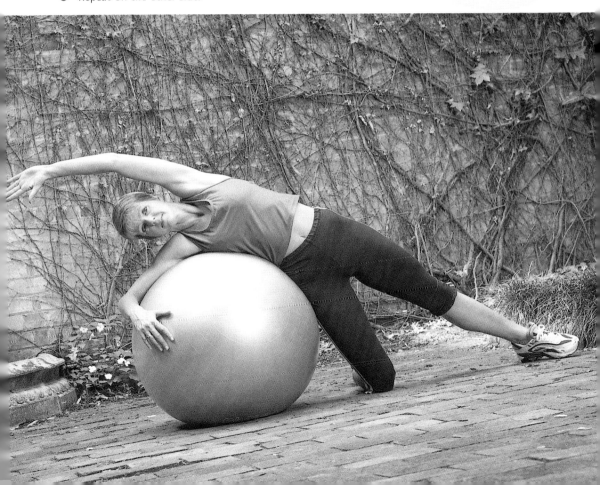

prone rotation

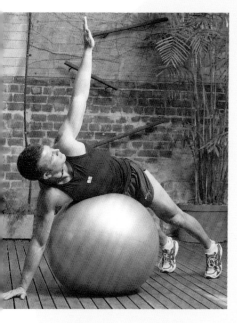

- Lie forward over the ball and rest your feet and fingertips on the floor.
- Gently raise and turn to reach one arm towards the ceiling.
- Repeat on the other side.

drape

- Lie foward over the ball and rest your feet and fingertips on the floor.
- Relax your neck and gently rock forward and back.

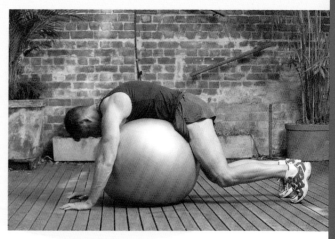

prone back extension

- Place your hands on the ball and slowly raise your chest up, gently extending your spine.
- Keep within your comfort range. You don't need to go into an extreme extension for the stretch to be effective.
- Hold for 40 to 60 seconds.

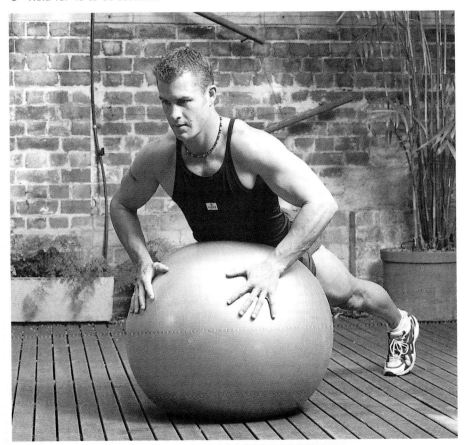

quads stretch

- Lie over the ball and place your left hand and foot slightly out to the side.
- Raise your right arm and leg off the floor.
- Reach around to hold your right ankle.
- Gently lift your leg to stretch the front of your right thigh.
- Hold for 40 to 60 seconds.
- Lower your hand and foot to the floor, roll across and repeat to the other side.
- If you are finding it hard to balance, place your supporting hand and foot a little further out to the side.
- Keep a little space between your foot and your butt to avoid stress through the knee.

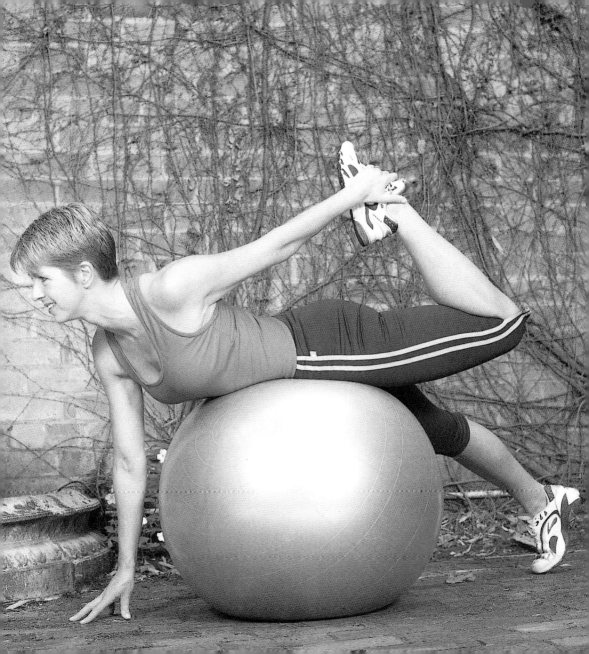

seated side stretch

- Sit forward on the ball with your feet wide apart.
- Roll the ball to the right, reaching your right hand up to the ceiling and stretching the right side of your body. Your right knee should be bent and your left knee straight.
- Roll the ball across to the left and repeat to the other side.
- Hold the side stretch for flexibility or roll from side to side to focus on mobility.

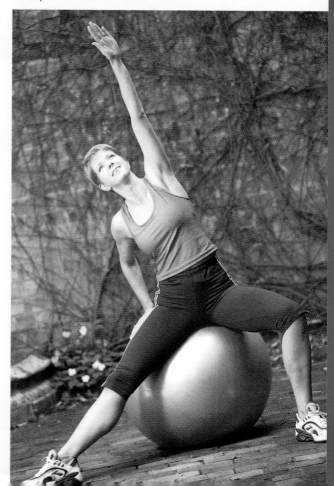

hip flexor stretch

- Sit foward on the ball with your feet wide apart.
- Stand up, turn sideways to the left then sit back down 'side-saddle' on your left butt.
- Sit upright and roll the ball forward to stretch the front of your right hip.
- Hold for 40 to 60 seconds.
- Stand up, turn to face the other direction and repeat to the other side.
- Make sure both feet are pointing in the same direction you are facing and keep your back heel off the ground.

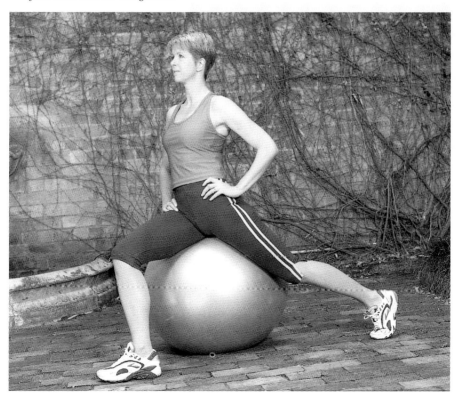

seated hamstring stretch

- Sit forward on the ball with your feet wide apart.
- Turn your body to look over one leg.
- Keep your back straight as you lower your chest towards that side.
- Roll the ball back gently to straighten that knee.
- Hold at the point of slight stretch for 40 to 60 seconds.
- Roll slightly further if you feel the hamstrings release.
- Bend your knee to roll back up.
- Repeat on the other side.

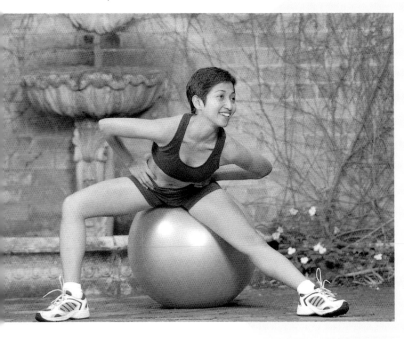

inner thigh stretch

- Sit forward on the ball with your feet wide apart and your hands resting on your thighs.
- Roll slowly to one side, then the other
- Hold for 40 to 60 seconds on each side for flexibility or roll slowly from side to side for mobility.
- You can perform this exercise sitting upright or leaning forward with your hands resting on the floor, depending on your flexibility.

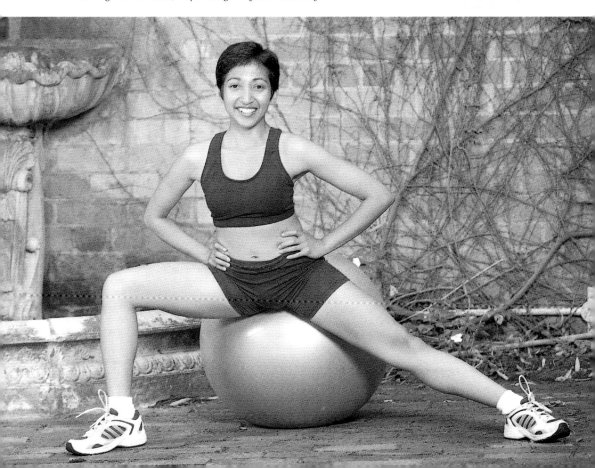

back and
butt stretch

- Sit forward on the ball with your feet wide apart.
- Keep your back straight and lean forward.
- Rest your elbows on your thighs or put your hands on the floor.
- Gently roll the ball back to increase the stretch in your back, thighs or buttocks.
- Hold for 40 to 60 seconds and then slowly roll back up.

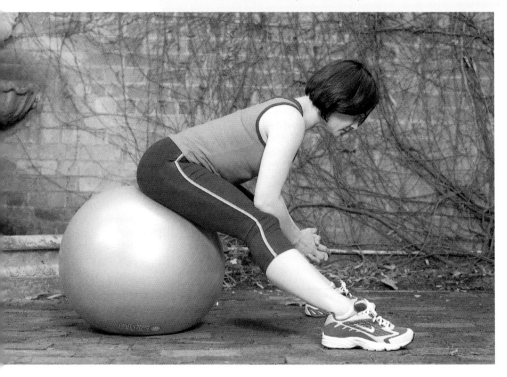

upper back stretch

- Sit forward on the ball with your feet wide apart and your hands resting on your thighs.
- Keep your back straight and lean forward.
- Wrap your hands behind your calves to hold your shins.
- Pull gently upwards against your arms to stretch across your upper back.
- Hold for 40 to 60 seconds.
- Release your arms and place your hands on your thighs to return to an upright posture.

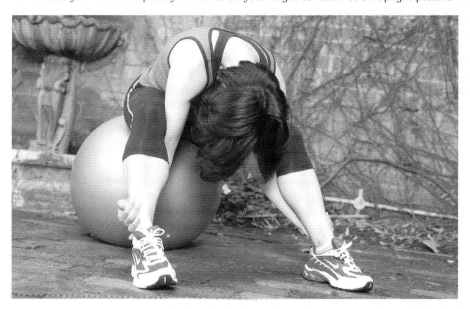

hip circles

- Sit on the ball and slowly roll the ball and your hips in a circle.
- 3 to 5 circles in each direction.
- Don't rush— the slower, the better to relax and release your back.

triceps stretch

- Sit tall on the ball.
- Reach your left hand towards the ceiling, then bend the elbow to take your hand down to the back of your neck.
- Use your right hand to gently push the elbow down.
- You should feel a stretch in the triceps at the back of your left arm.
- Hold for 40 to 60 seconds.
- Repeat on the other side.

neck and shoulders stretch

- Sit tall on the ball with your feet hip-width apart and your arms relaxed by your sides.
- Tilt your right ear to your right shoulder then walk the fingers on your left hand further down the ball to lower the left shoulder.
- Hold for 40 to 60 seconds.
- Roll your shoulders up, back and down x 3.
- Repeat on the other side.

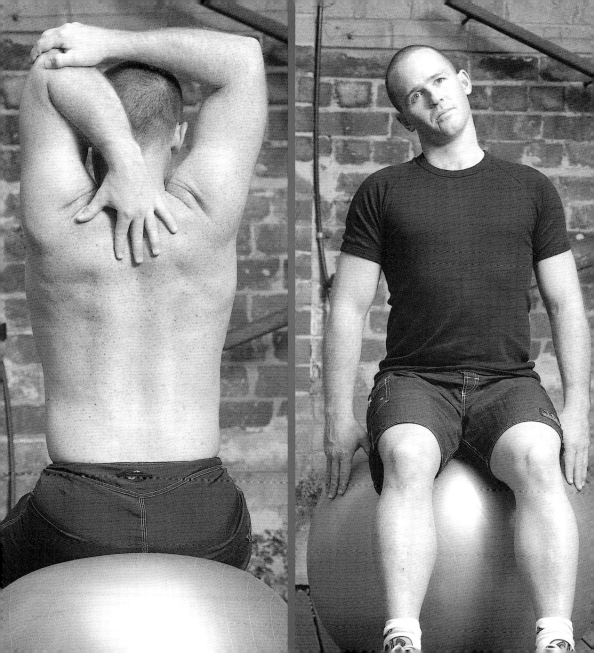

back extension stretch

- Sit tall on the ball with feet hip-width apart.
- Slowly roll from the sitting position until your elbows and then your upper back are on the ball.
- Allow your back to gently arch back over the ball.
- Support your neck at all times.
- Hold for 40 to 60 seconds.
- Roll up slowly, using your elbows to help.
- For a longer back extension stretch, straighten your legs and roll back.

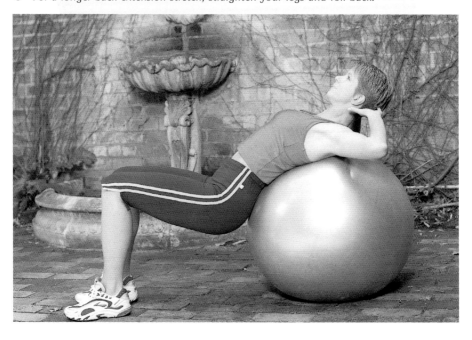

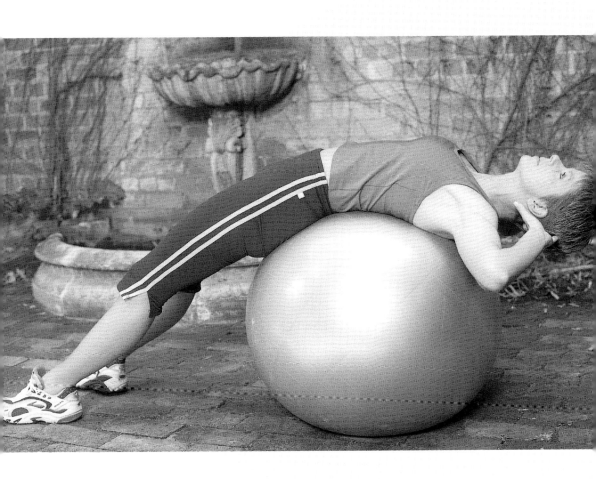

163

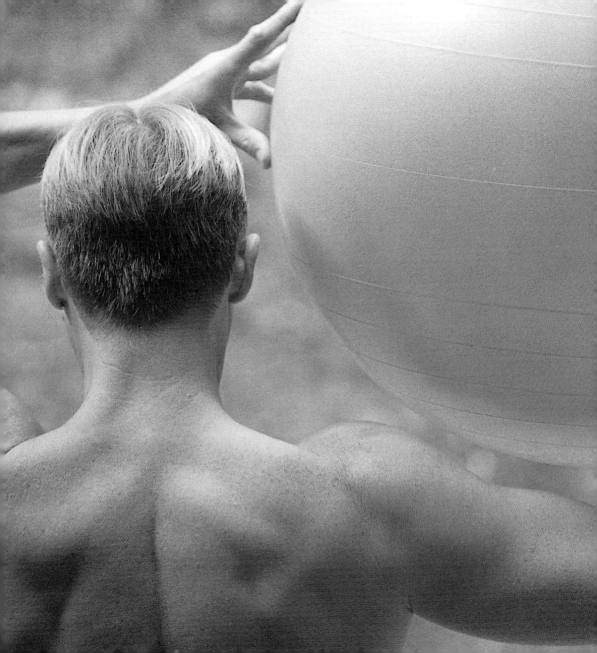

The exercises in **Strong to the core** can be combined in an endless number of ways to suit your training goals. Or you can save time and effort by selecting one of the training programs.

The programs range from gentle 'getting started' sessions through to intense core stabilisation drills and include strength workouts that target specific body parts. There are prenatal fitness, back care and rejuvenating flexibility programs, so there is something here for everyone.

The programs can be performed on their own or combined with cardiovascular exercise. Whether you are a veteran strength and conditioning expert or just starting out, remember to vary your training and reward yourself with the soothing and refreshing 'relax and release' sessions for a balanced, thriving body and a clear, calm mind.

The programs have been designed to deliver outstanding results, so - mix, match and enjoy!

training programs on the ball

all round workout I

getting started

A total body workout that is ideal if you are just starting out or looking for a light session. Start with the warm up on pages 32 to 35, and be sure to stretch appropriately after each exercise.

1
seated leg raise,
page 40

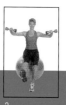

2
seated lateral
arm raise, page 42

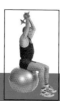

3
seated triceps
press, page 48

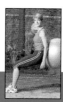

4
wall squat,
page 54

5
wall push-up,
page 62

6
abdominal curls,
page 82

7
side lean,
page 94

8
ball bridges,
page 68

9
wide row,
page 100

10
prone leg raise,
page 110

11
one leg lower,
page 128

12
kneeling back
stretch, page 145

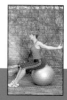

13
back and chest
stretch, page 35

14
neck and shoulders
stretch, page 160

all round workout 2

sensational all over strength and tone

A moderate strength session that works your body from top to toe. Start with the warm up on pages 32 to 35 and be sure to stretch appropriately after each exercise.

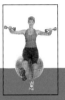

1
lateral arm raise,
page 42

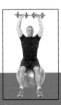

2
shoulder press,
page 44

3
wall squat with
bicep curls, page 56

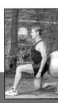

4
wall lunge,
page 58

5
chest press,
page 72

6
ab curls,
page 82

7
obliques,
page 84

8
roll away,
page 86

9
push ups,
page 120

10
side leg raise,
page 90

11
back extension,
page 108

12
triceps press back,
page 104

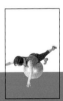

13
raise and reach,
page 116

14
hamstring lift and
roll, page 132

all round workout 3

the total body challenge

A tough, total body workout to challenge the experienced exerciser. Start with 30 minutes of cardio or perform the warm up on pages 32 to 35. Be sure to stretch appropriately after each exercise.

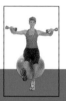

1
lateral arm raise
(add leg raise),
page 42

2
shoulder
press, page 44

3
seated row
(add alternating
leg raise), page 46

4
triceps dip,
page 50

5
wall squat
with bicep curl,
page 56

6
lunge with
upright row,
page 60

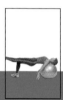

7
supine stability
(single leg option),
page 70

8
chest press (feet
together), page 72

9
flys (add
single arm fly),
page 74

10
lat pullover,
page 76

11
abdominal curls
(feet together,
walk 1 step back
over ball), page 82

12
roll away (roll
ball side to side),
page 86

13
side leg raise,
page 90

14
lateral curl,
page 92

15
wide row (add
alternating leg
raise), page 100

16
prone low row
(add alternating
leg raise), page 102

17
triceps press back,
page 104

18
prone swim kick
with one arm
raised, page 112

19
raise and reach
(three-limb
option), page 116

20
push up (longer
lever), page 120

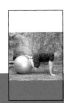

21
prone tuck,
page 124

22
hamstring lift and
roll, page 132

23
gluteal stretch,
page 141

24
spinal rotation,
page 142

25
kneeling back
stretch, page 145

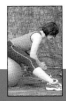

26
quads stretch,
page 152

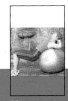

27
back and butt
stretch, page 158

28
back extension
stretch, page 162

great expectations

exercising for two

Safe and effective exercises for pre and post-natal fitness. Be sure to check with your health care provider before beginning any exercise program. Perform one slow pelvic floor contraction between each exercise (page 27).

1
hip circles,
page 34

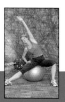

2
side reaches,
page 34

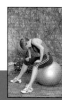

3
back roll,
page 35

4
back and
chest stretch,
page 35

5
seated leg
raise, page 40

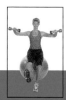

6
lateral arm raise
(weights 1 or no
weights), page 42

7
seated row
(weights 1 or no
weights), page 46

8
seated tricep press
(weights 1 or no
weights), page 48

9
wall squat,
page 54

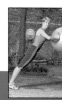

10
wall push up,
page 62

11
ball bridges,
page 68

Listen to your body. If any exercise causes discomfort, stop and seek professional advice. Remember that the health and safety of you and your baby is your top priority.

12
rock and roll,
page 144

13
kneeling
back stretch,
page 145

14
lats stretch,
page 146

15
pecs stretch,
page 147

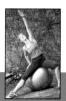

16
seated side stretch,
page 154

17
seated hamstring
stretch, page 156

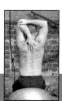

18
triceps stretch,
page 160

19
hack and butt
stretch, page 158

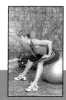

20
back roll,
page 35

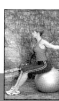

21
back and chest
stretch, page 35

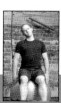

22
neck and
shoulders stretch,
page 160

back in action

keep your back strong, stable and injury-free

Use this program to improve the function of your spine and your quality of movement every day. If you suffer from back pain, seek assessment and advice before any exercise and do not use weights.

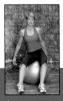
1
hip circles,
page 34

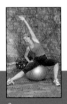
2
side reaches,
page 35

3
back and chest
stretch, page 35

4
seated leg raise,
page 40

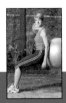
5
seated row,
page 46

6
wall squat,
page 54

7
wall push up,
page 62

8
side lean,
page 94

9
supine stability,
page 70

10
wide row,
page 100

11
prone push back,
page 106

12
raise and reach,
page 116

13
one leg lower,
page 128

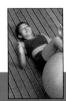
14
the clock,
page 130

relax your back

keep your back supple and mobile

Ease your body with these spinal stretches.

1
roll and reach,
page 138

2
gluteal stretch,
page 141

3
spinal rotation,
page 142

4
reach and release,
page 143

5
rock and roll,
page 144

6
kneeling back
stretch, page 145

7
lats stretch,
page 146

8
pecs stretch,
page 147

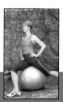
9
seated side stretch,
page 154

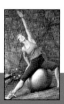
10
hip flexor stretch,
page 155

11
seated hamstring
stretch, page 156

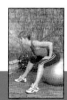
12
back roll,
page 35

13
back extension
stretch, page 162

14
neck and shoulders
stretch, page 160

backs, abs, butts and thighs

shape and definition where it counts

Use this program to sculpt a stronger midsection and below.

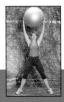
1
reach and squat,
page 32

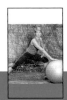
2
side lunges,
page 33

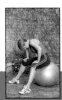
3
back roll,
page 35

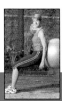
4
wall squat,
page 54

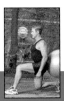
5
wall lunge,
page 58

6
supine stability,
page 70

7
flys (single arm),
page 74

8
lat pullover,
page 76

9
ab curls,
page 82

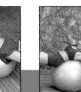
10
oblique curls,
page 84

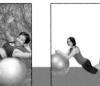
11
roll away,
page 86

12
side leg raise,
page 90

13
lateral curl,
page 92

14
wide row,
page 100

15
back extension,
page 108

16
prone swim kick,
page 112

17
pike,
page 114

18
plank,
page 122

19
hamstring lift and
roll, page 132

20
spinal rotation,
page 142

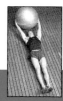
21
reach and release,
page 143

22
lats stretch,
page 146

23
kneeling back
stretch, page 145

24
gluteal stretch,
page 141

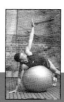
25
prone rotation,
page 150

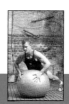
26
prone back
extension,
page 151

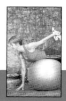
27
quads stretch,
page 152

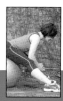
28
back and butt
stretch, page 158

chest and upper back

well balanced and strong

Build a well-balanced, strong upper body for fabulous definition and tall, proud posture.

1
back and chest
stretch, page 35

2
seated row,
page 46

3
chest press,
page 72

4
flys,
page 74

5
lat pullover,
page 76

6
wide row,
page 100

7
prone low row,
page 102

8
prone push back,
page 106

9
push up,
page 120

10
kneeling back
stretch, page 145

11
pecs stretch,
page 147

12
upper back stretch,
page 159

13
lats stretch,
page 146

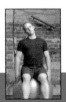
14
neck and shoulders
stretch, page 160

abs and back

honing in on your midsection

A challenging abdominal workout that focuses equally on back strength
to sculpt your midsection.

1
back and chest
stretch, page 35

2
lat pullover,
page 76

3
ab curls,
page 82

4
oblique curls,
page 84

5
lateral curl,
page 92

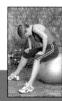

6
roll away,
page 86

7
wide row,
page 100

8
back extension,
page 108

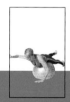

9
prone swim kick,
page 112

10
raise and reach,
page 110

11
prone back
extension,
page 151

12
lats stretch,
page 146

13
kneeling back
stretch, page 145

14
back roll,
page 35

arms and shoulders

square your shoulders to the world

Use this arm and shoulder program to give you strong,
defined arms and show-off shoulders.

1
lateral arm raise,
page 42

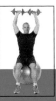

2
shoulder press,
page 44

3
seated row,
page 46

4
bicep curls; seated
or with wall squat,
page 56

5
chest press,
page 72

6
wide row,
page 100

7
prone low row,
page 102

8
triceps press back,
page 104

9
prone push back,
page 106

10
push up,
page 120

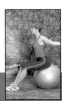

11
back and chest
stretch, page 35

12
pecs stretch,
page 147

13
triceps stretch,
page 160

14
neck and shoulders
stretch, page 160

thighs and gluteals

for a tough drill below the belt

Get on the ball for shapely legs and a butt of steel.

1
reach and squat,
page 32

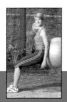

2
wall squat,
page 54

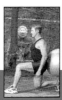

3
wall lunge,
page 58

4
side leg raise,
page 90

5
ball bridges,
page 68

6
supine stability,
page 70

7
prone leg raise,
page 110

8
prone swim kick,
page112

9
pike,
page 114

10
hamstring lift and
roll, page 132

11
hamstring stretch,
page 140

12
gluteal stretch,
page 141

13
quads stretch,
page 152

14
back and butt
stretch, page 158

core control I

fine tuning inner strength

A gentle core stability workout for injury prevention and a healthy spine.

1
hip circles,
page 34

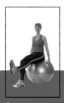
2
seated leg raise,
page 40

3
wall push up,
page 62

4
ball bridges,
page 68

5
supine stability,
page 70

6
side lean,
page 94

7
raise and reach,
page 116

8
one leg lower,
page 128

9
the clock,
page 130

10
hamstring lift and
roll, page 132

11
spinal rotation,
page 142

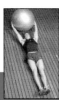
12
reach and release,
page 143

13
rock and roll,
page 144

14
back roll,
page 35

core control 2

strong to the core

An intense combination to challenge strength and stability of the shoulder girdle, pelvic girdle and spine.

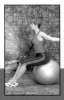
1
back and
chest stretch,
page 35

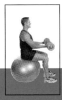
2
seated row
(add leg raise),
page 46

3
triceps dip,
page 50

4
flys (single arm),
page 74

5
supine stability
(leg raised off the
floor), page 70

6
roll away,
page 86

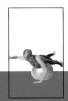
7
prone swim kick
(one hand off the
ground), page 112

8
plank,
page 122

9
prone tuck,
page 124

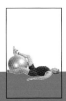
10
one leg lower
(arms across
chest), page 128

11
hamstring lift and
roll (arms reaching
up above chest),
page 132

12
spinal rotation,
page 142

13
lats stretch,
page 146

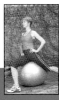
14
hip flexor stretch,
page 155

relax and release 1

roll up to unwind

Perform this series of movements and stretches with slow, calm breathing
to relax your body and mind.

1
supine rock,
page 138

2
adductor stretch,
page 138

3
hamstring stretch,
page 140

4
gluteal stretch,
page 141

5
spinal rotation,
page 142

6
reach and release,
page 143

7
lats stretch,
page 146

8
pecs stretch,
page 147

9
kneeling side
stretch or extended
side stretch, page
148 and page 149

10
hip flexor stretch,
page 155

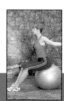

11
back and
chest stretch,
page 35

12
back roll,
page 35

13
back extension
stretch, page 162

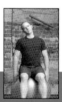

14
neck and shoulders
stretch, page 160

relax and release 2

long muscles and increased mental focus

Minimise injury and maximise well being with this relaxing combination.

1
rock and roll,
page 144

2
kneeling back
stretch, page 145

3
prone rotation,
page 150

4
drape,
page 150

5
prone back
extension,
page 151

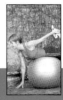

6
quads stretch,
page 152

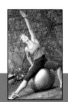

7
seated side stretch,
page 154

8
seated hamstring
stretch, page 156

9
seated inner thigh
stretch, page 157

10
back and butt,
page 158

11
upper back stretch,
page 159

12
triceps stretch,
page 160

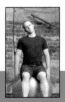

13
neck and shoulders
stretch, page 160

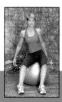

14
hip circles,
page 159

acknowledgements

A friend once told me, it takes far more than an author to write a book. She was right! So many wonderful people have played a role in this one.

It is one thing to have a great idea, but it is another to make it happen. So, thank you to Jill Brown, Commissioning Editor, ABC Books, for orchestrating the transformation of a dream into a reality. Her time, expertise and patience have been invaluable. And thank you to Liz Dene for bringing us together.

Thanks too to Jon Reid, the whiz behind the lens, and designer Ingo Voss for his creative style and flair in bringing the words and pictures together so perfectly on the page.

Thank you to Fitball Therapy and Training Australia, especially Alison and Arthur, for many exciting years together, sharing the evolution of ball training in fitness.

There are many others to thank: The wonderful and very patient models: Steve Brossman, Jill Brown, Shannon Ponton (Hard'N Up Personal Training), Carol Dutton and Keith Donald.

Annette Alison for her excellent work on the introductory section.

The Australian Barbell Company.

The Mushroom Group of Companies for the use of their premises for the photo shoot at such a reasonable rate.

And then, of course, there are the numerous friends, physiotherapists and fitness leaders who have educated, inspired or simply supported me.

I am so lucky to have a caring and encouraging family, without whose help (and child care) this would have been tough to complete.

Dave, Dan and Jess come last and yet they matter most. Thank you for your patience and love and allowing me to explore ideas beyond motherhood.

about the author

In 1994 Lisa Westlake left her career as Senior Physiotherapist in the Road Trauma Intensive Care Unit at the Alfred Hospital in Melbourne to increase her work and involvement in the fitness industry. She was Australian Fitness Leader of the Year in 1999 and 2000. She is Director of Physical Best, a company that develops specialist exercise programs, including the Australian fitball program. She is Instructor trainer for Fitball Australia here and in Asia. She lectures at the School of Physiotherapy at Melbourne University and for the course in Human Movement at Deakin University, and presents courses and workshops for physiotherapists and fitness professionals. She is a popular and well-regarded presenter at national and international fitness conventions, such as those for the Australian Physiotherapy Association, the Chiropractors and Osteopaths of Australia, Australian Fitness Network and Asiafit. She contributes articles to Ultrafit, Me and Women's Health magazines and Network magazine (the magazine for the fitness industry). She has produced five videos on fitball training.